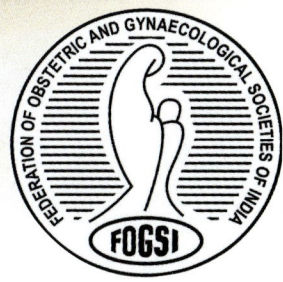
Federation of Obstetric and
Gynaecological Societies of India

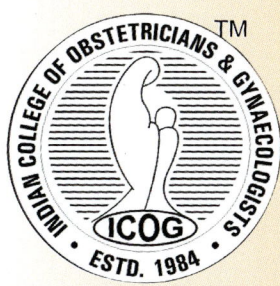
Indian College of Obstetricians
and Gynaecologists

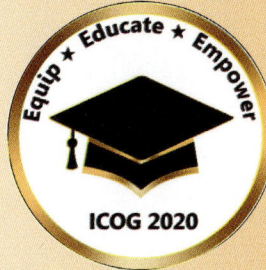
ICOG 2020

PET
Prevention, Examination and Treatment of Domestic Violence and Sexual Assault Cases

PET
Prevention, Examination and Treatment of Domestic Violence and Sexual Assault Cases

Chief Editor

Mandakini Megh MD DGO FICMCH FICMU FICOG
Chairperson ICOG-FOGSI
International Vice President, MWIA Central Asia
Consulting Obstetrician and Gynecologist
Director, Dr Megh's Gynaeo Care (a specialized clinic for women and adolescent girls)
Dean, Indian College of Medical Ultrasound (former); Vice President, FOGSI (2012–13)
Head, Cama and Albless Hospital (former); Deputy Director, Government of Maharashtra (former)
RCH, Family Welfare, World Bank, Maternal Health Consultant, UNICEF; Past President, IFUMB

Co-Editor

Reena J Wani MD FRCOG FICOG DNBE FCPS DGO DFP
Professor and Unit Head, Department of Obstetrics and Gynecology
HBT Medical College and Dr RN Cooper Municipal General Hospital
Ex-Professor (Addl), I/C Family Welfare Program, Department of Obstetrics and Gynecology
TN Medical College and BYL Nair Ch Hospital, Mumbai
Chairperson, FOGSI, Perinatology Committee, 2015–2017
Core Committee Member, FOGSI, Violence Against Women Cell
Managing Committee Member, MOGS, UNESCO Bioethics
President, MBPC (Mumbai Breastfeeding Promotion Committee)
Section Editor, TIP; Peer Reviewer, JOGI

Assistant Editors

Kruti Doshi MBBS MS DNB FMAS
Obstetrician and Gynecologist and Endoscopic Surgeon
Speciality Medical Consultant
HBTMC and Dr RN Cooper Hospital, Mumbai

Preeti Deshpande MS (OBGY)
Consultant Obstetrician and Gynaecologist
Raheja-Fortis Hospital, Guru Nanak Hospital, Fellowship Infertility, Mumbai
Advanced Endoscopic Training, IRCAD (France)

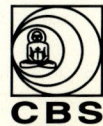

CBS

CBS Publishers & Distributors Pvt Ltd

New Delhi • Bengaluru • Chennai • Kochi • Kolkata • Mumbai
• Hyderabad • Jharkhand • Nagpur • Patna • Pune • Uttarakhand

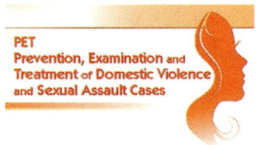

PET
Prevention, Examination and Treatment of Domestic Violence and Sexual Assault Cases

ISBN: 978-93-90709-37-3

Copyright © Federation of Obstetrics and Gynaecological Societies of India and Publisher

First Edition: 2021

Published by Satish Kumar Jain and produced by Varun Jain for

CBS Publishers & Distributors Pvt Ltd

4819/XI Prahlad Street, 24 Ansari Road, Daryaganj, New Delhi 110 002, India
Ph: 011-23289259, 23266861, 23266867   Fax: 011-23243014   Website: www.cbspd.com
                                                                e-mail: delhi@cbspd.com; cbspubs@airtelmail.in.
Corporate Office: 204 FIE, Industrial Area, Patparganj, Delhi 110 092, India
Ph: 011-4934 4934   Fax: 011-4934 4935   e-mail: publishing@cbspd.com; publicity@cbspd.com

Branches

- **Bengaluru:** Seema House 2975, 17th Cross, K.R. Road, Banasankari 2nd Stage, Bengaluru 560 070, Karnataka, India
  Ph: +91-80-26771678/79   Fax: +91-80-26771680   e-mail: bangalore@cbspd.com
- **Chennai:** 7, Subbaraya Street, Shenoy Nagar, Chennai 600 030, Tamil Nadu, India
  Ph: +91-44-26680620, 26681266   Fax: +91-44-42032115   e-mail: chennai@cbspd.com
- **Kochi:** 42/1325, 1326, Power House Road, Opp KSEB, Power House, Ernakulam 682 018, Kochi, Kerala, India
  Ph: +91-484-4059061-65/67   Fax: +91-484-4059065   e-mail: kochi@cbspd.com
- **Kolkata:** 6/B, Ground Floor, Rameswar Shaw Road, Kolkata 700 014, West Bengal, India
  Ph: +91-33-22891126, 22891127, 22891128   e-mail: kolkata@cbspd.com
- **Mumbai:** PWD Shed, Gala No. 25/26, Ramchandra Bhatt Marg, Next to JJ Hospital, Gate No. 2, Opposite Union Bank of India, Noorbaug, Mumbai 400 009, Maharashtra, India
  Ph: 022-66661880/89   e-mail: mumbai@cbspd.com

Representatives

• **Hyderabad**	0-9885175004	• **Jharkhand**	0-9811541605	• **Nagpur**	0-9421945513
• **Patna**	0-9334159340	• **Pune**	0-9623451994	• **Uttarakhand**	0-9716462459

Printed at Nutech Print Services, Faridabad, Haryana, India

to

*the nameless survivors who have suffered
domestic violence or sexual assault, and still have
surfaced like the Phoenix, rising from the ashes!*

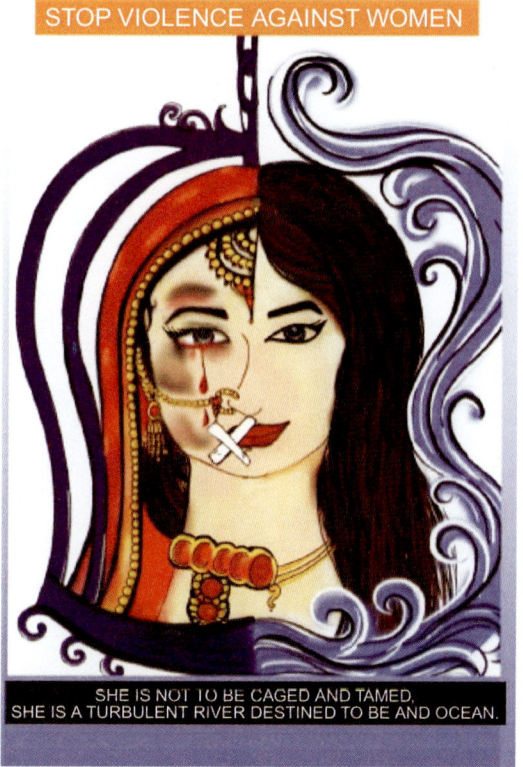

STOP VIOLENCE AGAINST WOMEN

SHE IS NOT TO BE CAGED AND TAMED,
SHE IS A TURBULENT RIVER DESTINED TO BE AND OCEAN.

Dr Teertha Shetty, Dr Roshni Khade

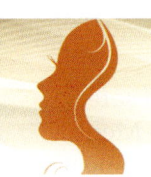

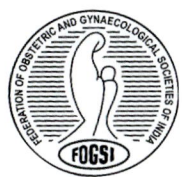 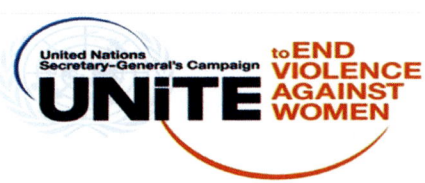

FOGSI invites you to make a difference!

Violence against girls and women has been prevalent since ages and across all civilizations. In India, the struggle for survival for a girl child begins right from the day she is conceived. We are a country of high maternal mortality and poor gender ratio. The skewed statistics reflect the underlying gender bias, the obsession for a male child, the patriarchy, and the social bigotry prevalent in our society.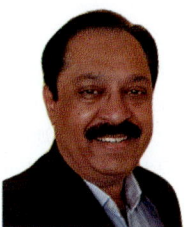

A woman in India can barely walk through a street without a nervous glance over a shoulder. Our dreams to call ourselves a progressive nation lies shattered by the NCRB (national crime records bureau) data. It states that the rape vulnerability of women has doubled over the last two decades. This is despite the statutory reforms that came into place post Nirbhaya. Every year thousands of women are victimised. The survivors suffer numerous indignities in their often futile attempts to get justice.

Violence against women and girls (VAWG) is not necessarily sexual, but the consequences are equally damaging. It has a profound impact on physical and mental health, with both immediate and long-term consequences. It also affects the social well-being of the women.

At FOGSI, we are a group of more than 38,000 gynecologists in the unique position to reach out to more than half of the 1.3 billion population of our country ... in fact to ALL since sensitization should be for men and women too! To raise awareness of violence against women; the United Nations General Assembly has designated November 25 as the International Day for the Elimination of Violence Against Women. The UN System's 16 Days of Activism against Gender-based Violence activities, from 25th Nov to 10th Dec took place under the 2020 global theme: *"Orange the World: Fund, Respond, Prevent, Collect*! In a unique initiative, this community connect E-conclave was conducted on 22/11/2020 from 9.30 am–8.30 pm and had about 21,000 viewers across different media including Facebook and Youtube. There were talks from experts in the field and interactive discussions to seek remedy to this grave problem. Results of essay and slogan competitions on the theme, to sensitise the community were released on that day. Our team has also released a booklet "KAVACH" on that day, for which Dr Reena Wani was instrumental in coordination and preparation.

"With Great Power comes Great Responsibility"—dear FOGSIANs, we have to rise to the occasion and translate good intentions into action, even if it may seem to be

a small step, to actually help someone at grassroots level, i.e. when our vision of safety for Indian women will become a reality!! I am very glad that Dr Mandakini Megh, Chairperson, ICOG-FOGSI and her team led by Dr Reena Wani have not only done a certified training workshop on this topic, but have also come out with this book which will be a ready-reckoner for all our members on all aspects of this subject.

Alpesh Gandhi
President, FOGSI

✍ *Editorial Note*

The various graphics in this section are the E-posters and physical posters prepared by junior doctors and nurses for 25th Nov 2020 competition arranged by the editorial team in HBTMC Cooper Hospital, Juhu, with prizes given by Mumbai Obstetric and Gynecological Society (MOGS) to increase awareness of this critical social issue.

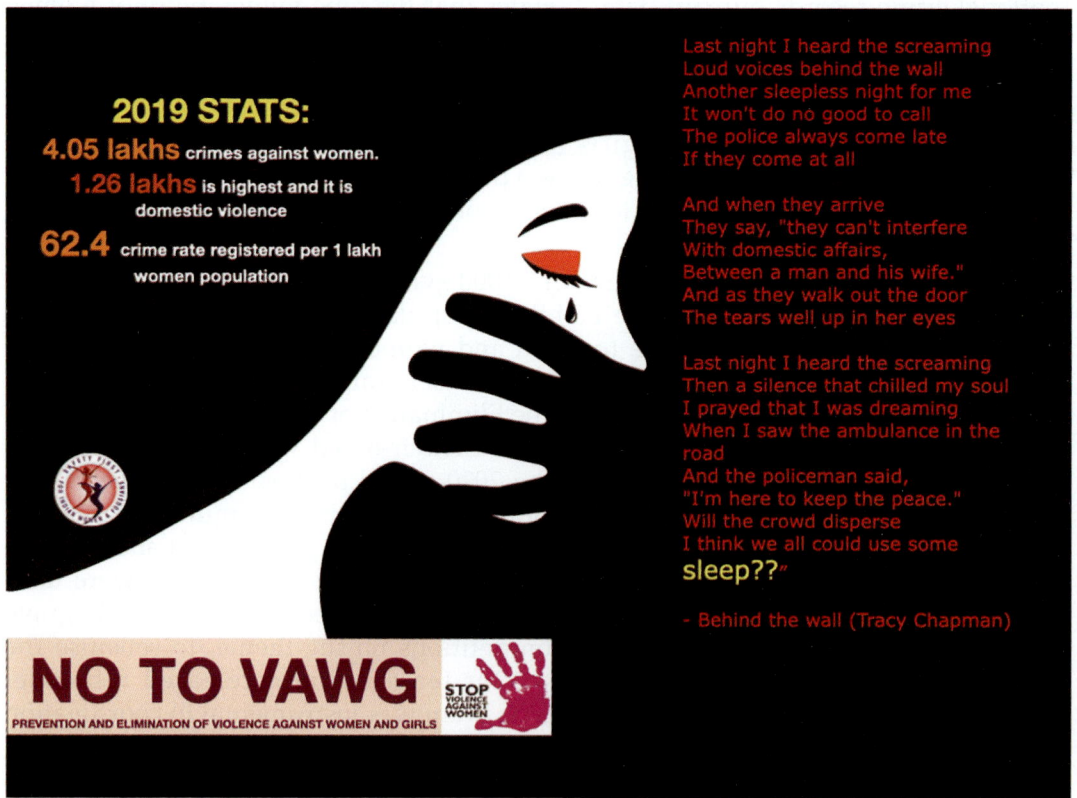

Dr Nivedita Pawar (1st Prize)

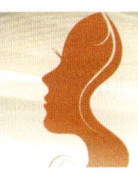

It is with great pleasure that I write the Foreword for an important publication that promises to make a difference to the practice of gynecology.

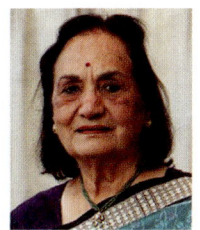

The title *PET: Prevention, Examination and Treatment of Domestic Violence and Sexual Assault Cases* is itself quite inclusive. It covers all aspects of the problem. It comprises approximately 27 chapters and has included practical as well as theoretical aspects.

For health care system to cater to this problem it is required to have a team of well trained professional with experience. Their approach has to be sensitive, perceptive and compassionate. One has to work with the long-term objective of giving solace and rehabilitation and maintain the dignity of the person.

We have worked on this issue for many years. Violence against women has many forms but has one thing in common that is, it is universal and is seen in all strata of society.

We have also interacted with United Nations which has taken a serious note of the rising incidence. Two of the experts from UN have contributed chapters to this book. Dr Padmini Murthy—MWIA's Representative to UN and Dr Bettina Pfleiderer—MWIA Past President have both contributed significantly to the alleviation of this problem. The annual UN Conference on "Status of Women" has discussions on this subject and brings out suitable pamphlets and scientific papers. In most countries as also in India the problem is under played. The reported cases are much less than the actual numbers as most women shy away from reporting. Even in the reported cases, the conviction rate is abysmally low.

In India, the law, however has been proactive. Since the famous 'Nirbhaya' case many facilities have been provided to the women in distress and given them shelter and comfort.

I would like to appreciate the tremendous contribution of the Editors Dr Mandakini Megh, Chairperson, FOGSI–ICOG and Dr Reena Wani and their team for their efforts in conducting a certificate course on this subject. This book is a compilation from lectures given by experts, which will help practitioners to give comprehensive care.

If the knowledge gained from this book translate into good clinical practice and helps some women who are in distress the authors will feel that they have not toiled in vain.

We live in interesting times. The future holds many opportunities to strengthen health systems for women and children. New partnerships will develop between Gynecologists, Social Workers, Members of Legal Profession, Public Health and Research Workers. Global players will come in with financing and administrative strategies and policies. In a sense, the world will come together and learn to live with "Gender Harmony".

Congratulations and best wishes to the authors, publishers and all those who have contributed to this magnificent production.

Happy reading and best wishes

Usha B Saraiya
MD DGO FIAC FICOG FRCOG (UK)
Past President of FOGSI and ICOG (2002)
Past Chairperson of ICOG (2006–2009)

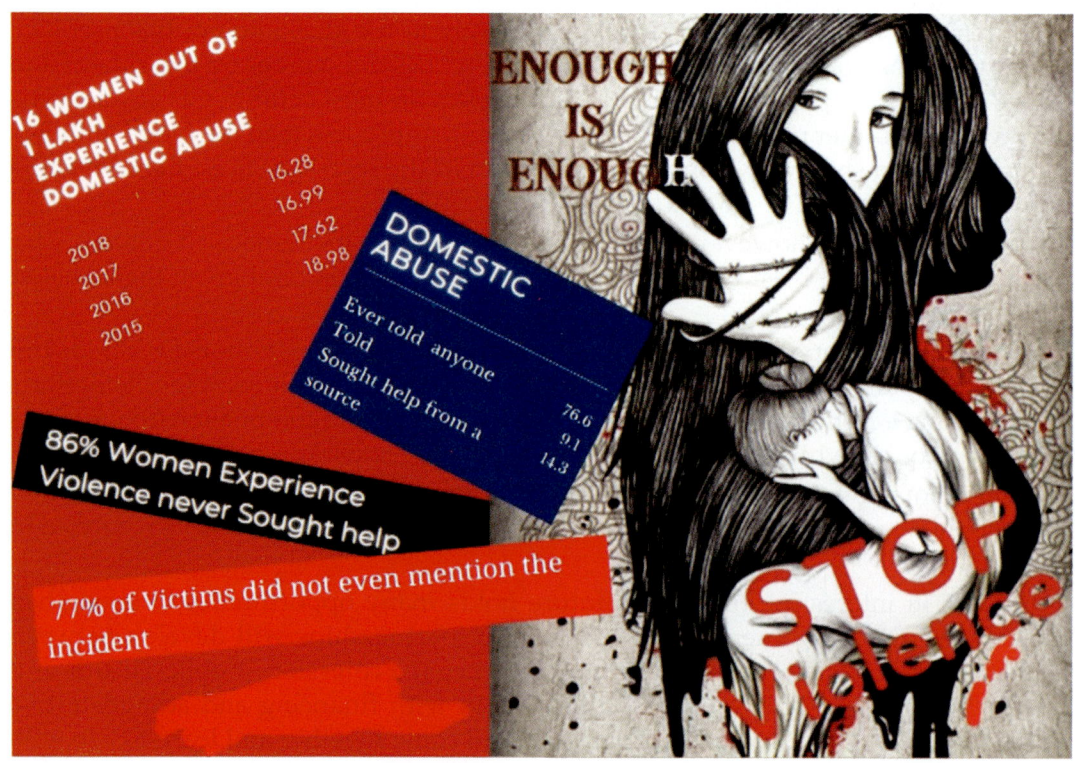

Dr Prashant Telharkar (2nd Prize)

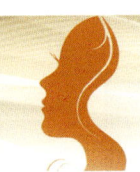

Dear FOGSIANs,

I am very happy to present to you the important work that Dr Mandakini Megh, Chairperson, FOGSI–ICOG and her team has created for you.

Sexual violence is a serious public health and human rights problem with both short- and long-term consequences on women's physical, mental, sexual, and reproductive health. According to NRCB data 2019, 88 cases of rape were reported every day in India; which is likely to be just the tip of the iceberg as a fraction of women who are raped file a complaint fearing social stigma.

The physical, financial and social vulnerabilities of women are fundamentally harmful to the future of any society. Violence against women is a crime. Not redressing these vulnerabilities fails to prevent harm to subsequent generations, and contributes to continuing the cycle of violence.

There is a need for wider awareness of the magnitude of the problem of violence against women. Only if this problem is recognized can it be addressed. Physicians, as advocates for women, are uniquely placed to assist in this. There is therefore a duty for professional societies and physicians to publicize information about the frequency of types of violence against women, and the implications for the wider society of allowing this to continue.

Physicians and the health care system can contribute to a great deal in all the three levels of prevention of VAW; which includes creating awareness about violence, identification of violence, providing acute care and long-term rehabilitation of survivors. This requires a team of trained and experienced, tender, sensitive, perceptive, and receptive health care providers who could deliver long-term mental health support and rehabilitation.

As a medicolegal and ethics person, I would like to appreciate Dr Mandakini Megh, Chairperson, FOGSI–ICOG and Dr Reena Wani and their team for their efforts in conducting a workshop on PET–VAW for practitioners. This book which is a compilation from multidisciplinary experts of OBGYN, psychiatrist law enforcement and NGOs; which will help practitioners to handle medico-legal cases.

Sanjay Gupte
Past President, FOGSI
Chairman, FIGO Committee for
Ethical and Professional Aspects of
Human Reproduction and Women's Health

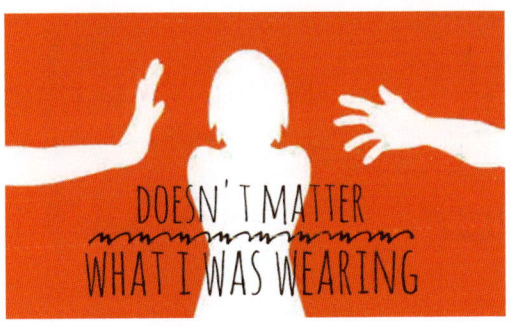

Dr Virendra Sutar

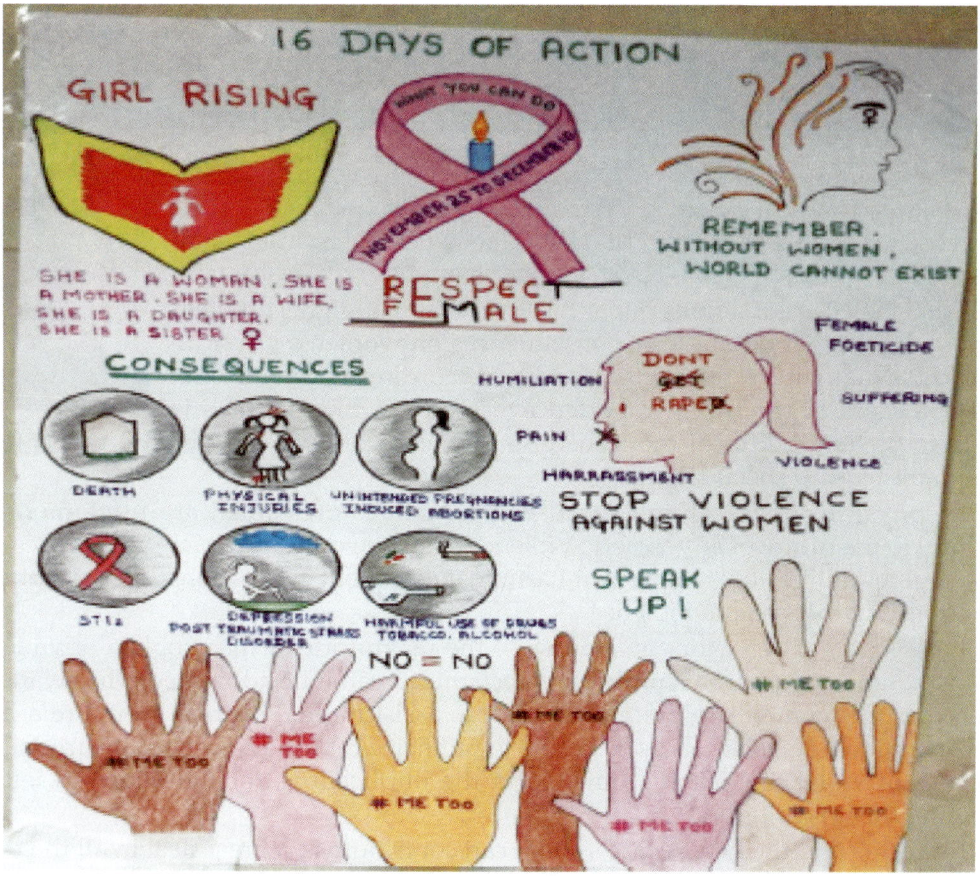

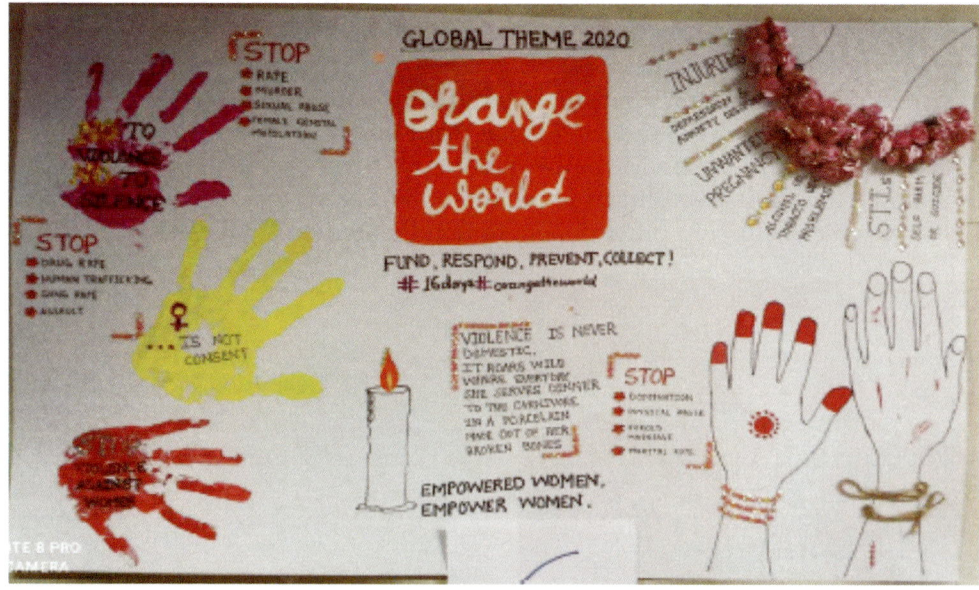

Dr Poonam Gowda (1st Prize TIE)

Dr Sumaya, Dr Yashshree, Dr Sukeshini (1st Prize TIE)

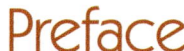

Preface

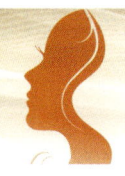

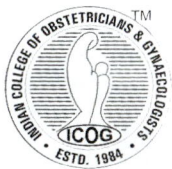 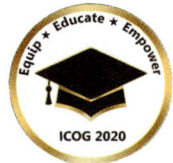

Theme of the Chairperson, ICOG 2020–2021
EQUIP_EDUCATE_EMPOWER

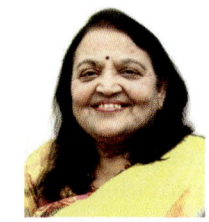

MD, DGO, FICMCH, FICMU, FICOG
Chairperson, ICOG

Greetings and Regards!

It is a privilege for me to write the Foreword for *PET: Prevention, Examination and Treatment of Domestic Violence and Sexual Assault Cases*. We are addressing the problems and challenges of very critical social issue of grave importance of today dealing with domestic violence and sexual offences. It is a proud feeling that this publication will help in every step to us, the medical professionals.

"If we are to fight discrimination and injustice against women, we must start from the home for if a woman cannot be safe in her own house then she cannot be expected to feel safe anywhere."

As we are aware domestic violence, sexual assault affects all parts of society, the responses that arise to combat it are comprehensive, taking place on the individual, administrative, legal, and social levels.

Keeping in mind, how to the prevent, doing examination and treatment of domestic violence and sexual assault cases, the articles have been compiled in this book. With the help of this book health professionals can use the guidelines as a day-to-day service document and/or as a tool to guide the development of health services for victims of sexual violence. The guidelines can also be used to prepare in-service training courses on sexual violence for health care practitioners and other members of multidisciplinary teams.

The guidelines will be useful for a range of professionals who provide care for victims of sexual violence: Health service facility managers, medico-legal specialists, doctors and nurses with forensic training, district medical officers, police surgeons, gynaecologists, emergency room physicians and nurses, general practitioners, and mental health professionals. These guidelines are meant to be adapted to specific local and national circumstances, taking into account the availability of resources and national policies and protocols. This book would be of much help to update knowledge and guide to deal with the situation in time.

In conclusion, I would like to quote the Israeli historian and scholar of the Holocaust; **"Thou shalt not be a victim, thou shalt not be a perpetrator, but above all thou shalt not be a bystander."**

As a chief editor of book along with co-editor Dr Reena Wani bring this very important and useful publication, *PET: Prevention, Examination and Treatment of Domestic Violence and Sexual Assault Cases*. We are sure this book will help you all in your day-to-day practice.

Wishing you a very happy and healthy coming year.

Dr Mandakini Megh
Chairperson, ICOG

Message from Co-Editor

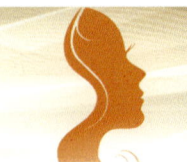

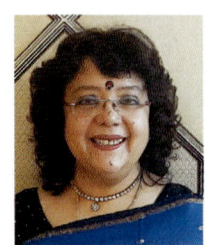

"We must be the change we want to see in the world" said Mahatma Gandhi.

We are the torch-bearers for women's health and are responsible for them from "Womb to Tomb" being often the primary health providers especially for women who never reach out to the health care system until they get have period problems or get pregnant. Hence, we are often in the privileged position of being first responders in situations of violence against women and children ... but the tragedy is that often the person hesitates to open up, or we fail to do what we should.

Violence against women and girls is a gross violation of human rights and remains largely unreported dues to impunity enjoyed by the accused, and a culture of shaming and blaming the victim. Despite Nirbhaya, Kathua and Hathras incidents, every day there are news reports of domestic and sexual violence. Intensive awareness drives and concerted efforts from every quarter is the need of the hour to quash this evil. It has been a neglected area of research, the available data are scanty and fragmented but after the #MeToo movement, more focus has been put on this area.

Often the health care system is blamed for not responding in a timely or appropriate manner when a girl or woman approaches for help or reporting. Often there is lack of clarity about procedure and protocols to be followed, or hesitancy on behalf of private sector to be involved.

The training workshop by ICOG–FOGSI was conceptualized by us to attempt to plug the gaps in knowledge and improve practices in dealing with violence against women and girls. The book was born out of the effort to collate information in concise form which can be referred to by each of you in times of doubt.

Our pledge and Hippocratic Oath requires us to rise to the challenge of "Saying no to Violence Against Women and Girls" ! If each one of us is able to help even one person, by reporting/facilitating/rehabilitating in a small way, we would have made a difference.

This is just the beginning, but we hope that it will show light at the end of the tunnel.

In the words of Sir Robert Frost

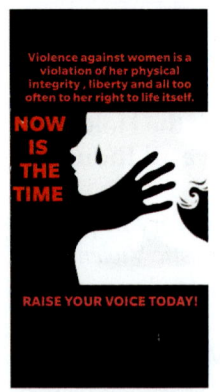

"The woods are lovely, dark and deep
But I have promises to keep
And miles to go before I sleep,
miles to go before I sleep ... ."

Reena J Wani
Co-Editor and Convenor, FOGSI–ICOG, PET Workshop
Core Committee Member, FOGSI, VAW Cell 2015–2021

Dr Sayesha Patel (1st Prize TIE)

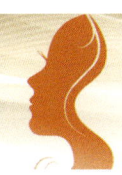

According to National Crime Records Bureau 2019 report, over 32000 women were raped in India, a number which has been steadily rising by 31% in the last decade. The first point of contact for victims of sexual assault are health care providers and the law enforcement. Health care professionals have a dual role to provide the survivor with the required medical and psychological treatment as well as to assist in their medico-legal proceedings.

Doctors in both public and private sectors are hesitant to take up cases of violence against women due to lack of clarity on examination and reporting. Hence, FOGSI–ICOG conducted an online 3-day certificate course and lecture series on prevention, examination and treatment (PET) of domestic violence and sexual assault cases.

The course was the brainchild of ICOG Chairperson Dr Mandakini Megh and Dr Reena Wani. The course coordinators were Dr Hema Relwani, Dr Kruti Doshi and Dr Preeti Deshpande.

With a multidisciplinary panel comprising of 15+ speakers from OBGYN, psychiatry, law enforcement, medico-legal experts and NGOs, the course was an immense success. It was attended by 574 delegates from public and private sector and received highly positive feedback for the practical approach discussed for dealing with domestic violence and sexual assault cases. At the end of the 3 days, 142 attempted and passed the online examination and got certification from FOGSI–ICOG.

In order to summarize the learnings from the course, FOGSI–ICOG is publishing this book on violence against women—prevention, examination and treatment (PET) which is aimed to be a handy manual for practitioners. We are glad to be part of this team preparing this important compilation of up-to-date information shared by our experts.

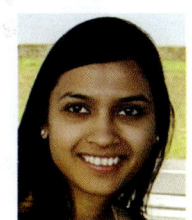

Kruti Doshi
Assistant Editor

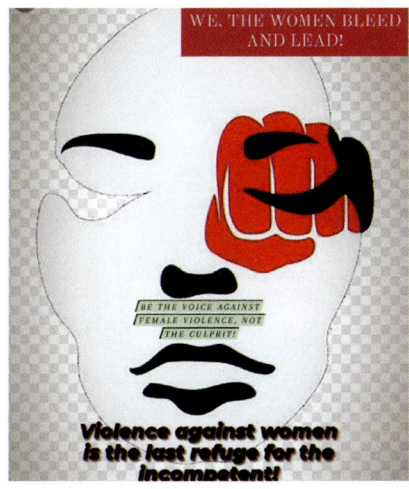

Dr Priyadarshini Dutta (3rd Prize TIE)

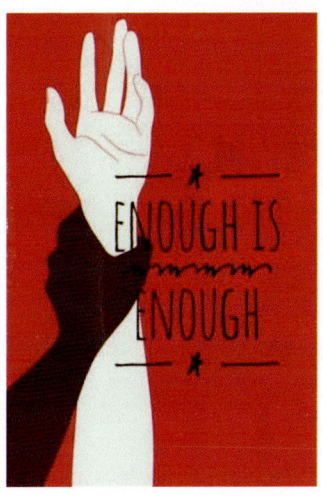

Dr Priyanka Surodwar

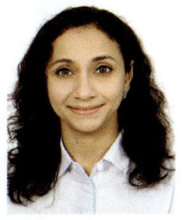

Preeti Deshpande
Assistant Editor

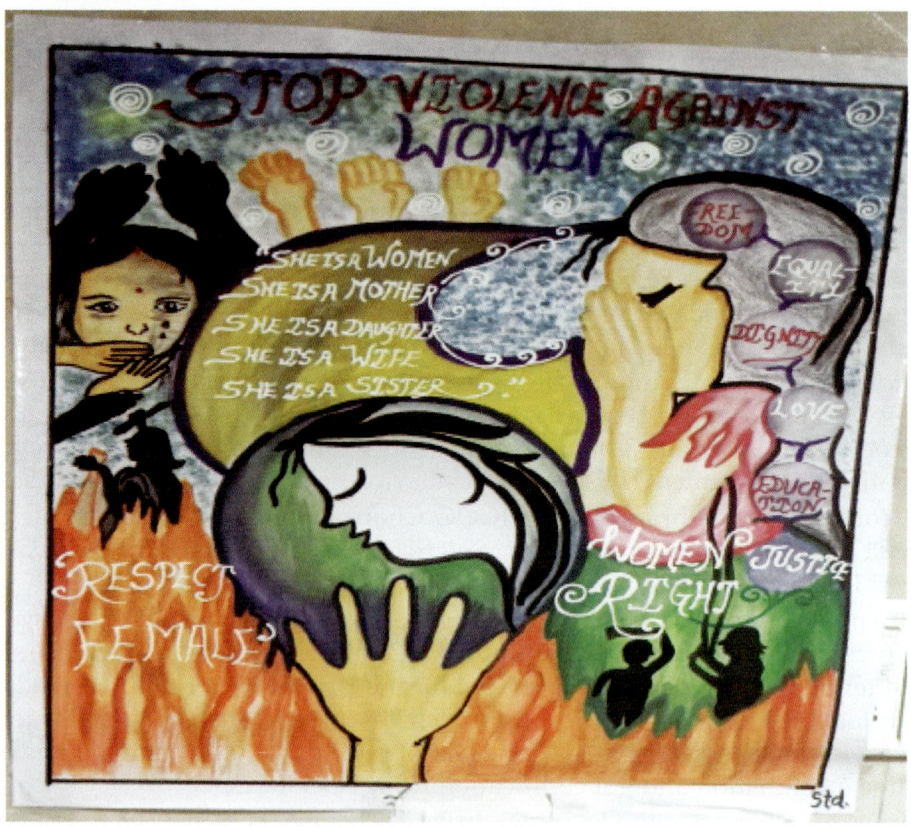

Student Nurse Divya Save (2nd Prize)

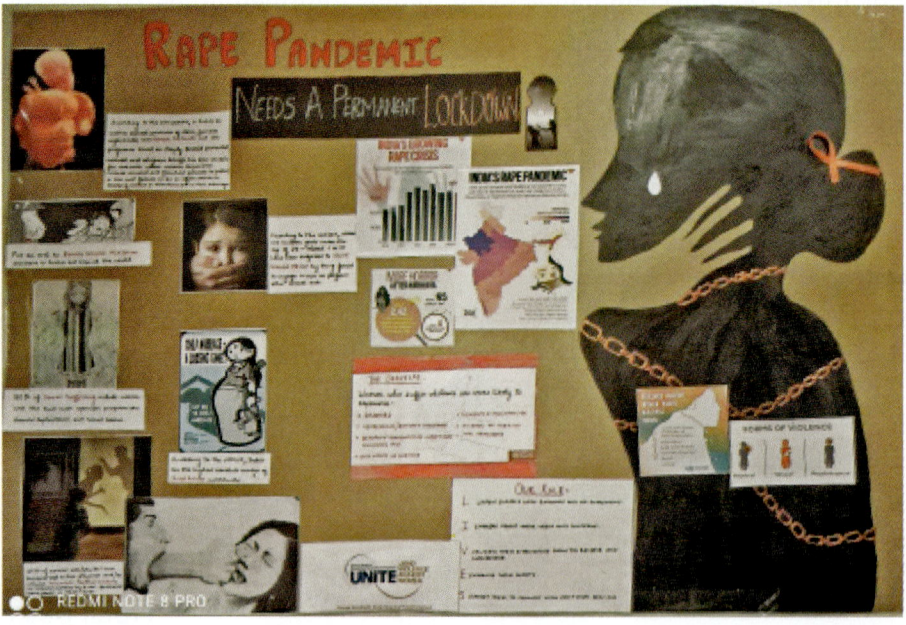

Dr Neha Mathews (3rd Prize)

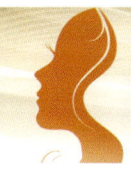

Acknowledgements

The editorial team would like to thank the following persons without whom this book would not have been possible.

- FOGSI President Dr Alpesh Gandhi for his vision and mission "Say no to Violence against Women and Girls".
- Our PET workshop coordinators and faculty who made it happen, despite the Corona Pandemic.
- ICOG office staff, especially Mrs Neelima More, and team of CBS Publications for their timely cooperation and efforts.
- Our spouses, without whose cooperation and adjustment of family time, we (ladies) could not have finished this project in time.
- Our family members ... Special mention of Mr Gorakh Megh, Dr Jatin Wani, Mr Anukool Deshpande and Mr Vinit Shah for being the men behind the strong women.
- A heartfelt thanks to each one of you who made it possible to publish this very important and timely release of the book *PET: Prevention Examination, Treatment of Domestic Violence and Sexual Assault Cases*.

Mandakini Megh
Reena J Wani
Kruti Doshi
Preeti Deshpande

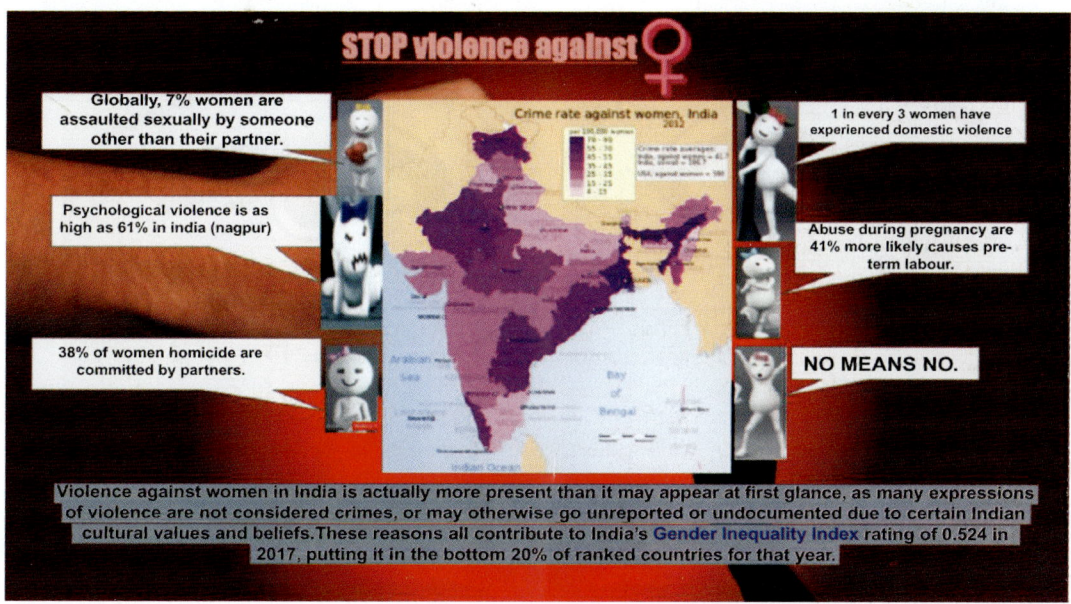

Dr Anjali Mulchandani, Dr Teertha Shetty, Dr Roshni Khade

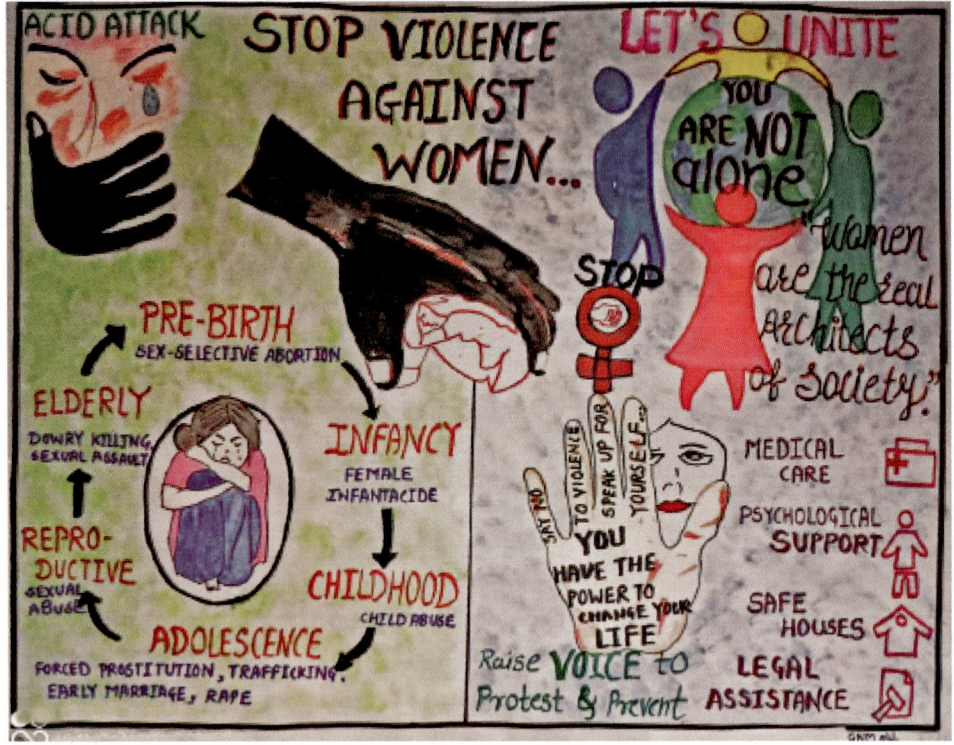

Student Nurse Mittal Vasave

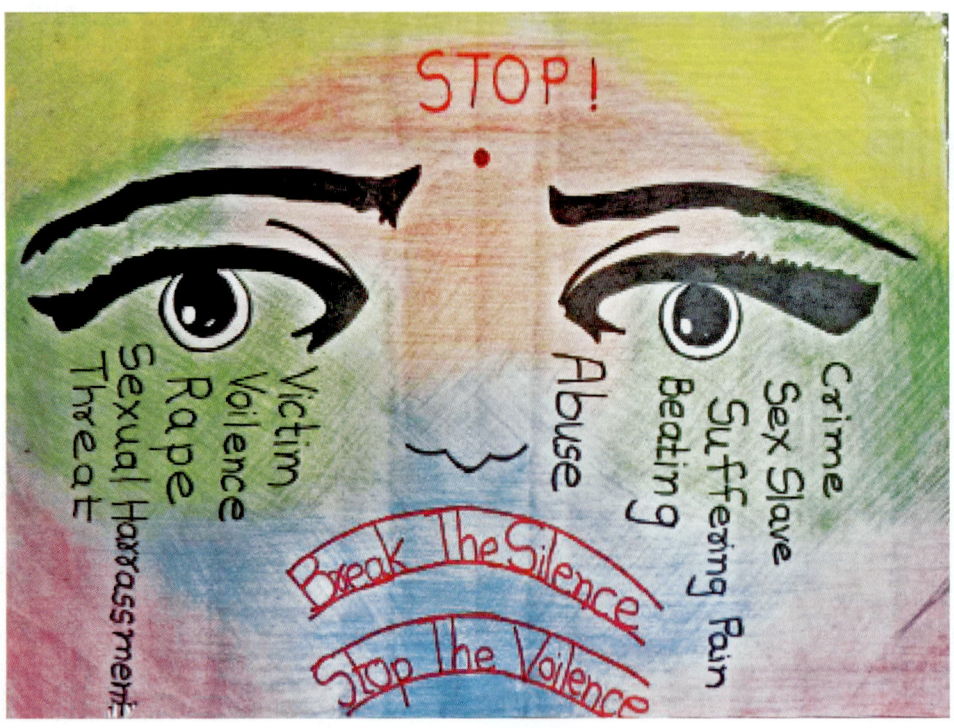

Dr Ramyata Parkhi

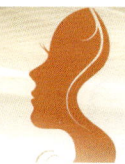

List of Contributors

Amit Karkhanis
Advocate, Corporate Advisor and
Medicolegal Consultant
Founding Partner of Kay Legal and
Associates LLP
Practising Medical Law for 20 years

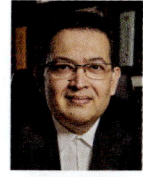

Arvind B Mulay DNB, DGO
Senior Resident
Department of Obstetrics and
Gynecology
HBTMC and Dr RN Cooper
Hospital, Mumbai

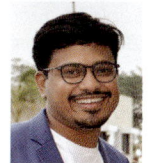

Bettina Pfleiderer PhD, MD
(Prof Dr med. Dr rer. nat.)
Clinic for Radiology and Medical
Faculty, University of Muenster
Albert-Schweitzer-Campus 1,
Building A1, 48129 Münster
Germany
E-mail: pfleide@wwu.de

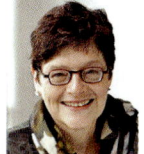

Bhavini Shah Balakrishnan
DNB, DGO
Director at Momma's Clinic
Awarded Dr Khurshed and Soonu
Sheriar Award by MOGS
Received Wonder Fogsian Award
by FOGSI

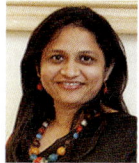

Hema Relwani MBBS, DGO, DNB
Assistant Professor
HBTMC and Dr RN Cooper
Hospital, Mumbai

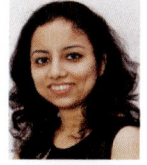

Jaydeep Tank
MD, DNB, DGO, FCPS, MICOG
Secretary Federation of Obstetrics
and Gynecological Societies of
India (FOGSI), Immediate Past
President Mumbai Obstetrics and
Gynaecology Society (MOGS)
Deputy Secretary Asia Oceania Federation of
Obstetrics and Gynaecology (AOFOG)
Chair International Federation of Obstetrics and
Gynecology (FIGO) Working Group on Safe
Abortion

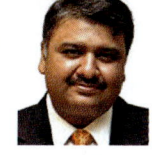

Jyothi Unni FRCOG
Director
Department of Obstetrics and
Gynecology Jehangir Hospital
Pune

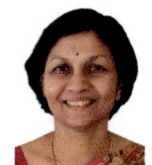

Jyoti Kukreja
BLS LLB Student of
Mumbai University
Interested in Medico-legal and
Consumer Laws

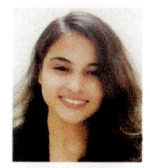

Kamaxi Bhate MD
Professor Emeritus, Community
Medicine, KEMH, Member
Secretary to 92 Internal
Committees, and Gender
Resource Centre of MCGM
2008–2019

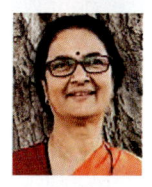

Kruti Doshi MBBS, MS, DNB, FMAS
Speciality Medical Consultant
HBTMC and Dr RN Cooper Hospital
Mumbai
Several Awards for Paper Presentation
at National Conferences

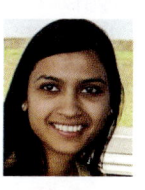

Mandakini Megh
MD, DGO, FICMCH, FICMU, FICOG
Chairperson, ICOG–FOGSI
International Vice President
MWIA Central Asia
Consulting Obstetrician and
Gynecologist
Director, Dr Megh's Gynaeo Care
Dean, Indian College of Medical Ultrasound (Former)
President, IFUMB 2004–2005
Vice President, FOGSI (2011–2012)
Supt and Head of Cama and Albless Hospital (Former)
Deputy Director of Government of Maharashtra
(Former)
RCH, Family Welfare, World Bank
Maternal Health Consultant, UNICEF
Clinical Training Incharge
Deputy Director Health Services, World Bank (MHSDP)
Recipient of MOGS "Shailaja Pandit" Award for
Working on "Woman Empowerment, Domestic
Violence, Contraception and Family Welfare
Recipient of DK Dutta Best Publication Awards
for FOGSI Books

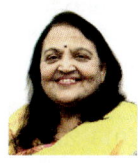
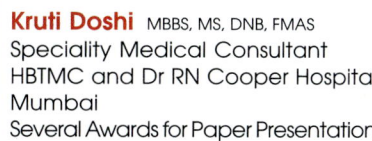

Meenakshi Deshpande

Consultant
Obstetrician and Gynaecologist
FOGSI VAW Cell-Master Trainer
FOGSI Repr. NIMC (PCPNDT,
MOHFW)
FOGSI—Member Ethics and MLC
Committee
IMA Pune Vice President, Chairperson IMA Pune
ML Cell, IMA MS.PC-PCPNDT Chairman
IMA Alt. CWC Member, Delhi HQ
E-mail: meenakshideshpande3@gmail. com

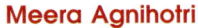

Meera Agnihotri

Professor and Head
Obst and Gynae
GSVM Medical College, Kanpur (Ex)
Presently Chairman, Ethics and
Research State Medical College
President WWW Foundation
Advisor: Women Health Cell Ministry of Health
Government of India

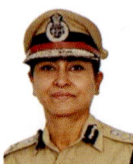

Meeran Borwankar

IPS, Author, Motivational Speaker, Advocate
IPS Maharashtra Cadre from 1981 to
till 2017
Publications on Investigation,
Gender, Law Enforcement,
E-Governance, Human Rights and
Community Participation

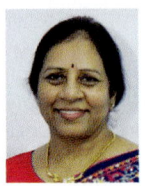

Meka Krishna Kumari

MD, DGO, FICOG
Professor, Apollo IMSR
Senior Consultant, Medicover
Hospitals
ICOG Governing Council Member
2018–2021

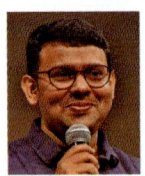

Milan Balakrishnan   MD, DPM, PGDM

Consultant Psychiatrist
Secretary, Bombay Psychiatric
Society
Associated with NGOs to Fight
Mental Health Stigma

Nayreen Daruwala

SNEHA
Program on Prevention of
Violence Against Women and
Children
E-mail: nayreen@snehamumbai.org

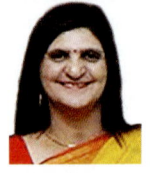

Nikhil D Datar

MD, DNB, FCPS, FICOG, LLB, DGO
Consultant Gynaecologist and
Health Rights Activist
Senior Obstetrician, Gynaecologist
and Medical Director
Cloudnine Group of Hospitals
Mumbai
Partner Lifewave Hospital LLP and Yashada Hospital
Founder President, Patient Safety Alliance
Recipient of Commonwealth Professional
Fellowship (2009–10) and Austrian American
Foundation Fellowship (2010–11)

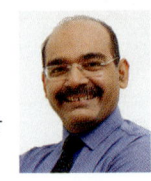

Padma Bhate-Deosthali

Senior Advisor, CEHAT
Consultant, Care India

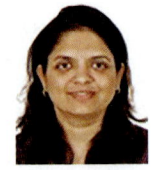

Padmaja Samant

MD, PGDBE, PGDHCM, FIME
Post Graduate in ObsGyn
at Seth GS Medical College
Mumbai
MUHS Task Force for Curriculum
Implementation
Founder Member and Coordinator
Division of Medical Humanities and Medical
Education Technology Unit at GS Medical
College, Mumbai

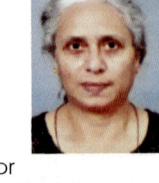

Padmini Murthy

MD, MPH, MS, FAMWA, FRSPH
Professor/Global Health Director
New York Medical College
First Indian Born American
Secretary General of MWIA in
100 Years
Global Health Lead American Medical
Women's Association
1st Indian American Recipient of Elizabeth
Blackwell Award in Over 70 Years
Delivered Dr Marie Catchatoor, Dr Jerusha
Jhirad and Dr Homi Collabawalla Orations
Chair International Health Section American
Public Health Association
Widely Published Multiple Platforms, Author and
Editor of 4 Books
Recipient of the Betha Van Hoosen Award from
AMWA for Service
Made Over 160 Presentations Nationally and
Internationally
Consultant to United Nations Population Fund,
Yoga Practitioner
Media Host and Presenter

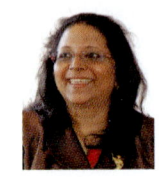

Paulina Juszczyk MA
Clinic for Radiology and Medical
Faculty University of Muenster
Albert-Schweitzer-Campus 1,
Building A11
48129 Münster
Germany
E-mail: paulina.juszczyk@wwu.de

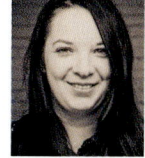

Preeti Deshpande
MS, FICOG, Fellowship Infertility
Advanced Endoscopy Training
(IRCAD), France
Consultant Obstetrician and
Gynaecologist
Winner of the Best Youth Council
Member Prize for 2 Consecutive
Years 2015–16 and 2016–2017
Member of Managing Council of MOGS 2019–20
Assistant Editor of the 2nd Edition of the Book—
Play By the Rules—an Update on Government
Policies, Regulation and Acts for Practicing
Obstetricians and Gynaecologists

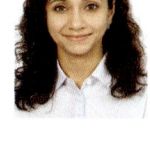

Rajshree Dayanand Katke
MD Obstetrics and Gynaecology, FMAS, FICOG
Professor and Head
Department of Obstetrics and
Gynaecology, Grant Govt.
Medical College and Sir JJ Group
of Hospitals, Mumbai,
Maharashtra, India, 400008
Ex-Superintendent, CAMA and Albless Hospitals
Mumbai, Maharashtra

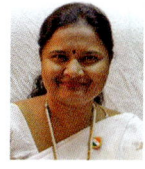

Rashmi Jalvee MS, DGO, DNB
Assistant Professor
Department of OBGY
HBT Medical College and Dr RN
Cooper Hospital, Mumbai

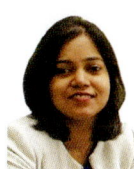

Reena J Wani
MD, FRCOG, FICOG, DNBE, FCPS, DGO, DFP
Professor and Head of Unit
Obstetrics and Gynecology
HBTMC and Dr RN Cooper
Hospital, Mumbai
Core Committee Member, FOGSI
Violence Against Women Cell 2014–2021
President, MBPC, Section Editor, TIP, Peer Reviewer,
JOGI
Chairperson, FOGSI, Perinatology Committee
2015–2017
Correspondence:
E-mail: reena.wani@rediffmail.com

Sachin Paprikar DGO
Senior Resident
Department of Obstetrics and
Gynecology
LBK Government Medical College
JGDP, CG
Ex-HBTMC and Dr RN Cooper
Hospital, Mumbai

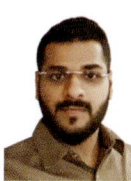

Sangeeta Rege
Director, CEHAT
Leads Initiatives for Health System
Response to Violence and
Integrating Gender Concerns in
Medical Education. Interested in
Gender, Medical Education,
Violence Against Women and Health Care
Published a Book for Routledge-Understanding
VAW/C-Understanding Responses and
Approaches in the Indian Health Sector (2020)

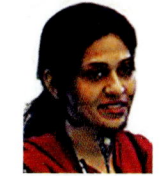

Sanjida Arora BDS
Research Officer with CEHAT
Principal Investigator to Assess
Prevalence of Domestic Violence
Amongst Pregnant Women during
ANC. Committee Member of
Anusandhan Trust's Institutional
Ethics Committee

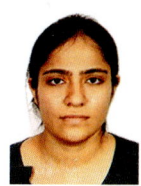

Shilpa N Naik MBBS, MD, PGDMLS
Academic Professor and Unit
Incharge, Department of
Obstetrics and Gynaecology
Byramjee Jeejeebhoy
Government Medical College
and Sassoon General Hospitals
Pune

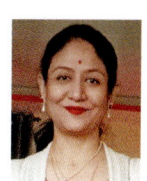

Vaishali Korde-Nayak
Master Trainer, FOGSI VAW Cell
(Violence Against Women)
General Secretary, POGS 2021–22
Professor and HOU, MIMER
Medical College, Pune
Senior Consultant, Critical Care
Obstetrics, Ruby Hall Clinic, Pune
E-mail: drvaishalinayak@gmail.com

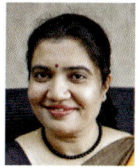

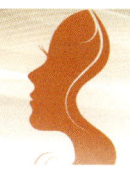

Contents

Section

I

Background and Epidemiology

Current Scenario of Sexual Violence

Vaishali Korde-Nayak

Sexual violence affects millions of women globally and its management had been out of the preview of health practitioners in the private sector. With the wide publicity of the Nirbhaya case in Delhi in December 2012, this issue has been brought center stage with a huge movement backed by political will. New laws have been brought into place with standardization of reporting and collection of medical evidence. All health providers are covered by these laws and it has become the responsibility of every doctor, whether in the public or private sector, to offer all medical support to the survivors of sexual abuse. Hence, it is important for doctors, especially gynecologists, to be updated and be aware of all legal, criminal, judicial, jurisprudence and health-related procedures, which will assist them in managing survivors of sexual abuse and also prevent themselves from facing difficulties with the law.

Definition of Sexual Assault, Related Acts and Laws

The World Health Organization (WHO) defines sexual violence as: "Any sexual Act, attempt to obtain a sexual Act, unwanted sexual comments/advances and Acts to traffic, or otherwise directed against a person's sexuality, using coercion, threats of harm, or physical force, by any person regardless of relationship to the victim on any setting, including but not limited to home and work.

The definition of rape (Section 375 of IPC)[1] as per the recent amendment (The Criminal Law (Amendment) Bill, 2013 as **passed by Lok Sabha on 19 March, 2013)** apart from peno-vaginal sexual intercourse includes other forms of sexual assault like oral penetration, urethral/anal penetration, fingering, use of objects (other than penis) for vaginal, urethral and anal penetration.

It also includes manipulation of any part of the body of a woman so as to cause penetration into the vagina, urethra, anus or any other part of body and application of mouth to the vagina, anus, urethra of woman and regards it as a 'rape' under the various circumstances explained in the law (for details please *see* Section II of Relevant Laws).

Section 354 of IPC deals with "criminal assault on a woman with intent to outrage her modesty" and Section 377 of IPC deals with "carnal intercourse against the order of nature". Immoral Traffic Prevention Act deals with human trafficking.[2]

WHO estimates that 150 million girls and 73 million boys under the age of 18 years are sexually abused every year.[3] Every second child is facing some form of sexual violence somewhere in the world!

The Important Terms

1. *Survivor* recognizes that the person is capable of taking decisions despite being victimized, humiliated and traumatized due to the assault. Use of the term survivor is important—believe the person and not pity her.
2. *"Victim"* is understood as a person who is not fully capable of comprehending situation at hand because of the victimhood faced, usually brought in by police. Victim also means a person is in need of compassion, care, validation, and support. The belief is that the person is so victimized that she may not be in a frame of mind to make decisions independently.
3. *Patient*, if a person comes on her own, term patient can be used.
4. *Accused* can be an adult or child. According to Protection of Children from Sexual Offences (POCSO) Act, 2012, any person both male and female, above the age of 18 years is an adult [IPC 2013]. Any person below 18 years, according to POCSO Act, 2012, is child.
5. *Sexual violence* is a significant cause of physical and psychological harm and suffering for women and children. Although sexual violence mostly affects women and girls, boys are also subject to child sexual abuse. Adult men, especially in police custody or prisons may also be subject to sexual violence, as also sexual minorities, especially the transgender community.

The perpetrators range from strangers to state agencies to intimate partners; evidence shows that perpetrators are usually persons known to the survivor.

Doctors have a dual role to play in terms of the Sexual Violence and Assaults and POCSO Act, 2012.

> *"Violence against women is perhaps the most shameful violation of human rights. It knows no boundaries of geography, culture or wealth. As long as it continues, we cannot claim to be making real progress towards equality, development and peace."*
>
> **—Kofi Annan, United Nations General, Assembly, New York, 5–9 June, 2000**

Culprits

More than 95% of sex offenders are relatives, neighbors, and friends. Hence, a majority of the cases go unreported.[3] Amongst those which are reported, 90% do not get justice because of lack of evidence.

Failure of Medical Profession

95% of victims do not get justice because doctors do not document correctly, nor do they collect the evidence correctly. The most important apathy of doctors is, the private sector of the medical profession does not want to get involved.

The two-finger test (TFT): Doctors still continue to use the 2-finger test as evidence. It is a judgemental and invalid test.

Widely performed across India, TFT checks the elasticity of a victim's vagina. A doctor gives his opinion on whether a woman is "habituated to sex" or not. Does that mean that "married women cannot get raped?" Does this mean that a woman who is in a consensual relationship deserves to be raped by others?

Most countries have scrapped it as archaic, unscientific and invasion of privacy and dignity.

In 1997, the law stipulated that only female doctors handle medical exam of rape victims.

In 2005, **ALL** registered medical practitioners (RMPs) were legally empowered to handle such cases.

These changes have introduced more physicians, to these sensitive examinations.

Problems in the Current Response of the Medical Profession to Sexual Assault to India

- Overemphasis on presence of injuries in medical examination. Absence of injuries interpreted as sexual assault did not take place.
- Poor history taking, nonrecognition of nonpeno-vaginal assaults.
- Mandatory police requisition for examination of sexual assault.
- Doctors attitudes—fear of appearing in court, avoidance, stereotypes about rape.
- Inadequate update on current situation that now it is **mandatory for all doctors approached by the survivor to collect evidence**.

Changes in the Acts after Nirbhaya

Amendments to the Indian Penal Code, Section 375 in 2013.[1]
- Expanded the definition of rape which also includes voyeurism, stalking, acid attacks and on proven guilty.
- Severe punishment of more than 7 years of imprisonment.

The POCSO Act, 2012

- The Protection of Children from Sexual Offences (POCSO) Act, 2012. It is applicable to whole of India and protects all children below 18 years from sexual harassment, sexual assault (penetrative and aggravated) and from using a child for pornographic purposes.
- Abetment or even an unsuccessful attempt to commit these offences are also punishable under the Act.
- Mandatory obligation to report the matter—media, hotel staff, hospital staff, clubs, photographic facilities, etc.
- Mandatory for police to register a FIR.
- Child's statement can be recorded at the child's home or place of his choice, preferably by a female police officer, not below the rank of sub-inspector.
- Amendments in the POCSO Act were passed in the Rajya Sabha on 24th July, 2019 including death penalty for aggravated sexual assault on children. Stringent punishment for other crimes against minors. Fines and imprisonment to curb child pornography.

The Manodhairya Yojana of the Maharashtra Government

- Initiated on 2nd October 2013, offers compensation to survivors of sexual abuse and acid attacks by the Government Amendment to the code of Criminal Procedure in 2009 that mandated state governments to have schemes for compensation of victims. Compensation—varies from ₹ 50,000 to ₹ 3 lakhs.
- Government to set up support services such as counseling, medical and legal aid.

FIGO Recommendation[4]

- Every gynecologist who is responsible for conducting medical forensic examinations should be trained, equipped and willing to present evidence in court of law. This is a duty towards sexually abused women, of all ages. Professionalism requires be discharged.
- If specialized rape crisis centers are unavailable, private locations should be provided.
- Consent needed to conduct medical forensic examination and all tests.
- While respecting their choice, doctors should stress advantages of this examination.

FIGO's priority is to address the barriers for clinicians to respond to violence against women through the use of advocacy, training and services.

How can we correct the present scenario?

- Training of medical students and sensitization of medicos.
- Change in medical (MBBS) curriculum by MCI/NMC. At least one question related to this subject should be included in the examination for undergraduate as well as postgraduate certification.
- To educate on uniform protocols for:
  - Examination of the victim
  - Collection of evidence
  - Referrals to other units
  - Management of the victim following abuse.

Violence Against Women

The United Nations defines violence against women as "any Act of gender-based violence that results in, or is likely to result in, physical, sexual, or mental harm or suffering to women, including threats of such Acts, coercion or arbitrary deprivation of liberty, whether occurring in public or in private life."[5]

Intimate partner violence refers to behaviour by an intimate partner or ex-partner that causes physical, sexual or psychological harm, including physical aggression, sexual coercion, psychological abuse and controlling behaviours.

Almost one-third (30%) of all women who have been in a relationship have experienced physical and/or sexual violence by their intimate partner. The prevalence estimates of intimate partner violence range from 23.2% in high-income countries and 24.6% in the WHO Western Pacific region to 37% in the WHO Eastern Mediterranean region, and 37.7% in the WHO South-East Asia region.[6]

Globally as many as 38% of all murders of women are committed by intimate partners. In addition to intimate partner violence, globally 7% of women report having been sexually assaulted by someone other than a partner, although data for nonpartner sexual violence are more limited.[6] Intimate partner and sexual violence are mostly perpetrated by men against women.

In May 2014, the Sixty-seventh World Health Assembly (WHA) adopted resolution WHA67.15 on "strengthening the role of the health system in addressing violence, in particular against women and girls, and against children." It requests the Director-General "to develop, with the full participation of Member States, and in consultation with United Nations organizations, and other relevant stakeholders focusing on the role of the health system, as appropriate; a draft global plan of action to strengthen the role of the health system within a national multisectoral response to address interpersonal violence, in particular against women and girls, and against children, building on existing relevant WHO work."[6]

The scope of the global plan of action is guided by resolution WHA67.15. The plan focuses on violence against women and girls, and against children, while also addressing common actions relevant to all types of interpersonal violence. It also addresses interpersonal violence against women and girls, and against children, in situations of humanitarian emergencies and post-conflict settings, recognizing that such violence is exacerbated in these settings.

CONCLUSION

Violence is preventable and is not inevitable. There is a need to address the economic and sociocultural factors that foster a culture of violence against women (VAW). Health care systems can reinforce interventions for prevention and management of gender-based violence particularly against women and girls. The health care system is the only institution that interacts with almost every woman at some point in her life and women living with violence are likely to visit health facilities more frequently than nonabused.

Interventions by health providers can potentially mitigate both the short- and long-term health effects of gender-based violence on women and their families.

REFERENCES

1. Central Government Act. Section 375 in The Indian Penal Code. https://indiankanoon.org/doc/623254/(accessed 02/01/2021).
2. MoHFW Guidelines and protocols: Medico-legal care for survivors/victims of sexual violence. 2013;23–7.
3. World Health Organization. Global status report on violence prevention 2014. https://www.who.int/publications/i/item/9789241564793 (accessed 02/01/2021).
4. Benagiano G. The role of FIGO in addressing violence against women: International journal of gynecology and obstetrics: 2002;78(1):S125–27.
5. World Health Organization. Violence against women. https://www.who.int/news-room/fact-sheets/detail/violence-against-women (accessed 02/01/2021).
6. WHO clinical and policy guidelines: Responding to intimate partner and sexual violence against women 2013.

Domestic Violence in COVID Crisis

Padmini Murthy

Abstract

The ongoing COVID-19 crisis has brought affected the global community in more ways than one. Not only has it resulted in the loss of millions of lives globally but has contributed to the dramatic rise in violence globally. Unfortunately, women are at greater risk of domestic violence and the silent pandemic as it is termed has increased during a pandemic especially during COVID. It is aptly as termed a shadow pandemic as many times the abuse is not evident to others but is present and is sometimes all pervasive, i.e. the girls and women in the family may be subject to ongoing Acts of violence. This chapter discusses the reasons why COVID-19 crisis has exacerbated domestic violence/gender-based violence (GBV) globally. The importance and positive outcomes of multi-sectoral approach in addressing DV/GBV during the current crisis will be mentioned in addition to highlighting examples of gender focused best practices in the context of addressing domestic violence globally.

Introduction

If we are to fight discrimination and injustice against women, we must start from the home for if a woman cannot be safe in her own house then she cannot be expected to feel safe anywhere.

Aysha Taryam

There has been a "horrifying global surge in domestic violence" since the start of the COVID-19 lockdowns, said United Nations secretary-general António Guterres in early April.

It is interesting to note the regional or global nature of despair associated with fear and uncertainty of pandemics provides an enabling environment that may exacerbate or spark diverse forms of violence against women including domestic violence. These which have described and documented an increase of violence against women during or post-pandemic are unfortunately scarce. On the other hand, media reports and anecdotal accounts of domestic violence are widespread. To illustrate this when the Ebola outbreak hit West Africa, an "epidemic" of "rape, sexual assault and violence against women and girls" was reported and this caused considerable collateral damage on many fronts.

Malaysia, for example, reported 57% more calls to domestic abuse helplines between 18 March and 26 March. Moreover, sexual and reproductive health clinics are closing worldwide.

In the United States, the National Domestic Violence hotline was proactive in releasing information in early March 2020 just as the pandemic started in the USA. The agency released a publication on "Staying Safe" during COVID-19, including anecdotal evidence of how perpetrators were using the virus as a scare tactic to threaten or isolate victims, and advising those at risk (i.e. women and girls) to have a safety plan, practice self-care and to reach out for assistance.[1]

Another challenge being faced globally is the closure of sexual and reproductive health clinics during COVID and lack of shelters for women to seek refuge as victims of domestic violence and this is a double burden they are facing.

Contributing Factors

Some of the contributing direct and indirect factors to domestic violence and gender-based violence globally are:[1]
1. Economic insecurity and poverty-related stress
2. Quarantine and social isolation
3. Disaster and conflict-related unrest and instability
4. Exposure to exploitative relationships due to changing demographics
5. Reduced health service availability and access to first responders
6. Inability of women to temporarily escape abusive partners
7. Virus-specific sources of violence (example mentioned above)
8. Exposure to violence and coercion in response efforts
9. Violence perpetrated against health care workers—especially female health care workers suffer a double burden in the homes and at work.

In addition, lack of gender equity and cultural practices which stifle women including mechanisms which deny women from expressing their opinion also contribute to the shadow pandemic, namely domestic violence/gender-based violence.

Challenges due to Pandemics including COVID-19

During the current and ongoing COVID crisis women have been affected disproportionately economically and socially.

Economic Hardship

According to a report released by the United Nations earlier this year, the crisis has precipitated disproportionally more layoffs among women, and this has impacted the rolling back of the slim gains made in female labor force. In addition, the economic hardship brought on due to the crisis has severely limited women's ability to support themselves and their families. Their hardships in many instances have further been compounded by the loss of employment of their male spouses or partners which has put them and their daughters at an increased risk for violence. The economic impact has been even more pronounced in female headed households as well.

Unfortunately, the current social protection systems and nets fall short and as mentioned in the brief, majority of women in S. Asia, sub-Saharan Africa, Latin America and The Caribbean work in the informal sector and in addition to facing an increased risk due to domestic violence do not have access to health care services.[2]

Health Challenges

In addition to economic hardships women have faced health challenges. For example, women may be at risk or exposure due to the occupational sex-segregation and it is important for the global community to note that 70% of health workers are women. Most of the nurses globally are women and have been the frontline workers during the current pandemic as are midwives, laundry workers and community health workers who have an increased risk of being exposed to the virus. They also often do not have access to personal protective equipment such as masks, caps, gloves, and gowns and this is another illustration of gender-based violence and domestic violence. To further illustrate this many women are not allowed to wear PPE by their male partners at home since the masks may be used by the men as women and girls are not considered valuable and disposable in many instances. Women continue to be shut out of global decision making and this impacts their reproductive and sexual health and general health as well. The UN policy brief further estimated that an additional 18 million women will lose regular access to modern contraceptives, given the current context of COVID-19 pandemics.[3]

There has been an increased incidence of unwanted pregnancies since girls cannot go to school due to crisis and the quarantine restrictions and many of them have been forced into early marriage by their parents. The pandemic has seen a rise in the number of unwanted teenage pregnancies, globally.

After the recent Ebola outbreak in Sierra Leone in 2014, some studies estimated that teenage pregnancies were 23% higher than in the previous year.[3]

For example, in Kenya authorities in the country have been registering thousands of additional cases of pregnant underage girls during the current pandemic. This is because they lack access to birth control and in many instances have been sexually abused often by strangers because of rape. In sub-Saharan Africa, a report released in October 2020 alone, 608,000 additional girls are thought to be at risk of child marriage, and 542,000 additional girls at risk of early pregnancy. As we are aware adolescent pregnancies have grave consequences for women's health. Teenagers are often at a higher risk for maternal morbidity and mortality. Which is even more exacerbated during the present. As mentioned earlier the number of girls dropping out of school has increased and one of the contributing factors has been pregnancy. This will have not only a short-term impact but a long-term impact as well.

Unfortunately female health care providers globally are at an increased of abuse when they give the patient or relatives news that the patient has tested positive for COVID and are often blamed. This is illogical as these frontline workers whether a physician, nurse or a laboratory technician give information about a positive test but are not responsible for the disease. This is an example of institutional violence and further contributes to the burden of violence against women which has resulted in "burn out" and exhaustion.

In addition to the physical injuries sustained because of women being in proximity with their male partners who are abusive they also experience severe mental trauma and often as already mentioned do not have access to the necessary support and health care services. Due to the lack of safety nets these women often have no where to go and are also at an increased risk for suicide. They are unfortunately unable to enjoy good health which according to the World Health Organization is a complete state of physical, mental, and social well-being. Often women and girls who are affected by COVID may be denied access to supportive treatment as often their lives due to the all pervasive gender inequality.

The lack of feminine hygiene products during the pandemic has been a major challenge. Girls and women do not have access to sanitary pads, tampons, and menstrual cups. Access to these products is further compounded by economic hardship, social restrictions, and lack of availability. Furthermore, girls and women with physical deformities and mental health issues who are often marginalized face even more challenges in access to feminine hygiene products.

Social Hardships

In addition, the lack of access to clean running water for women and the girl child is an illustration of gender-based violence/domestic violence. To illustrate this further the chore of fetching water is mostly regarded as the responsibility of the women or girls and during the pandemic this task has become even more challenging due to the risks of getting exposed to the virus or raped. Very often women and girls do not have the freedom to use the water they have brought, and this is another illustration of violence against women and girls since they are often forced to go out without protection in unsafe conditions during the pandemic. Restrictions due to gender norms being enforced, need to obtain permission to access health care services and not being able to access social support as they are often isolated and threatened by their abusers and since most of the male partners are at home due to quarantine or being unemployment the incidence of physical and emotional violence against women and girls increases. To sum up the various challenges faced by these women are many fold.

Tracking the Gender Impact of COVID-19

The use of a gender lens in tracking COVID-19 is a valuable tool in addressing the disproportionate effects of COVID. Unfortunately, at present the available data to track primary health effects by sex on cases and deaths is incomplete for most of the global population and is practically. Nonexistent for low income countries. It is also unavailable for reference even for health care workers, and the data is available only in a few handful of countries.

1. Countries such as the US which are affluent or rich and mid-incomes countries such as Brazil have not clearly reported infection rates by sex/gender (although they report deaths by sex).

2. The lack of recent data is a problem for most indicators to track secondary effects, as is the regularity with which they are reported since 2015 when the sustainable development goals were adopted the UN member states.

3. At present there is adequate data to track secondary health effects on maternal health and adolescent births, but ironically there is insufficient data to document effects of lack of access and the well-being of girls. The available data on women's mental health have adequate coverage and frequency but are based on estimates with large gaps in underlying data. This unfortunately is not an accurate picture as estimates are used.

4. The economic indicators often inadequate to track the secondary effects of the pandemic on economic well-being by gender. Neither job losses nor increases in unpaid care work by sex can be fully monitored with the available data. In contrast, sex-disaggregated education indicators are most abundant with available time series. One of the reasons could be lack of data on number of women working in the informal sector.

5. "Indicators like social protection coverage, personal ID coverage, and mobile phone ownership, which can monitor whether short-term mitigation measures exacerbate pre-existing gender inequalities, have been incorporated only recently into international data sets and have low coverage. This is a significant data gap in need of immediate attention."

6. "Gaps in frequency and timeliness for most indicators selected to track the gender effects of the pandemic are greater for rich than for poor countries, constraining rich countries' abilities to monitor the effects of the pandemic on gender inequalities."[4]

Examples of Best Practices Globally

1. Kenya and Trinidad and Tobago are making use of technology in their judiciary to address the issue of GBV.

2. Pharmacies and supermarkets in France and Spain are a part of a safety network and have put into place emergency warning systems to provide counseling services to victims of GBV and assist with reporting abuse during the current crisis.

3. In another move, almost 20,000 hotel rooms across France have been designated as safe spaces.

4. The police department in Odisha is using telephone services to reach out to those women who lodged complaints about abuse pre-COVID crisis.[2]

5. The United Nations Development Program (UNDP) in Somalia has partnered with local communities to implement neighborhood watch initiatives in local communities and to make them alert to any incidents of GBV in their area.

6. Similarly, in Mexico, UNDP, is working with another UN agency, namely UN women to use phones and online platforms to support vulnerable women via the LUNA centers, which have been created as safe spaces for women and girls.

7. In the Dominican Republic, UNDP and BHD Bank recently created a partnership to facilitate referral services of domestic violence cases that are reported by the bank's customers. This is a great illustration of public–private partnership in addressing the silent pandemic of GBV.

8. In addition, UNDP is coordinating with other UN sister agencies, development partners, and governments on Spotlight Initiative, a joint EU–UN partnership to end violence against women and girls. This global, multi-year initiative aims to assist 50 million direct beneficiaries across five regions and more than 25 countries.[2]

Recommendations by World Health Organization for health systems and abused women: Please refer to the enclosed **Figures 2.1** *and* **2.2.**

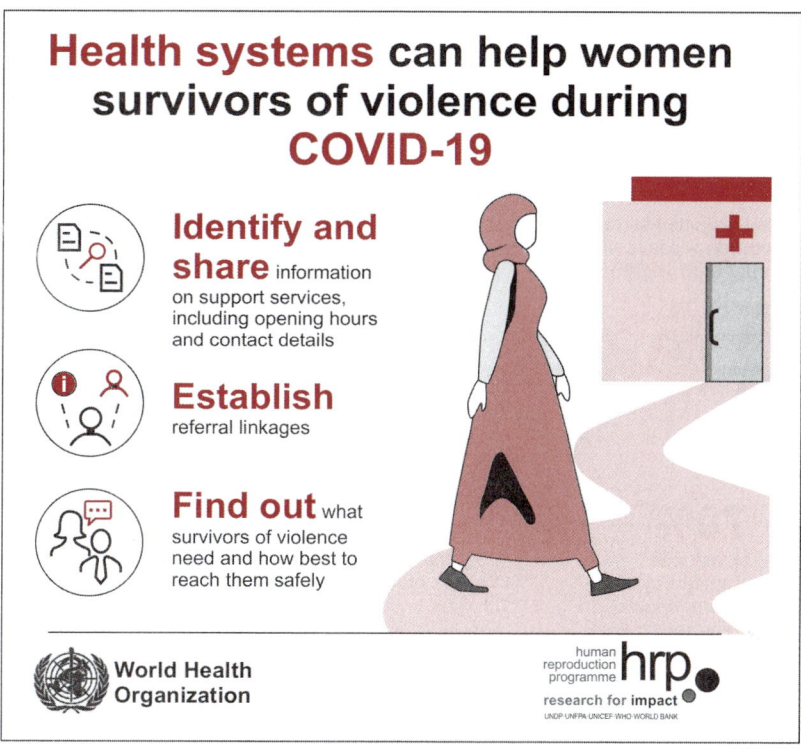

Figure 2.1: WHO recommendations

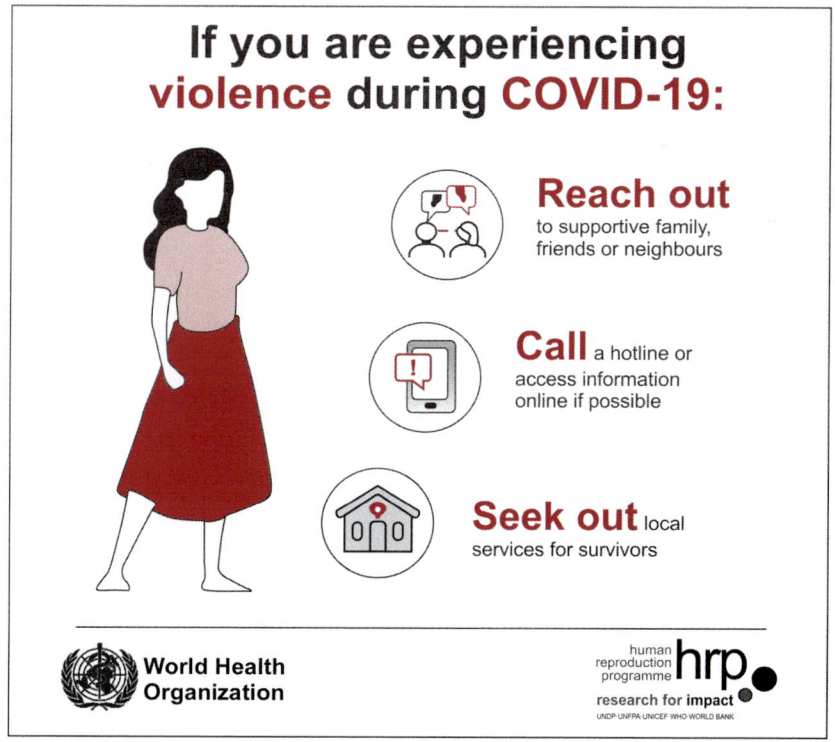

Figure 2.2: WHO recommendations

Double Pandemic: Please refer to the enclosed Figure 2.3.

A Double Pandemic

Gender-based violence in Latin America and the
early experience of women during COVID-19

The United Nations estimates that
1 in 3 women will face violence
during **their lifetime.**

Latin America has the **highest** rates of
gender-based violence in the **world.**

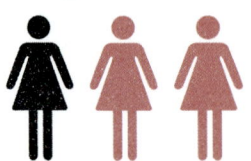

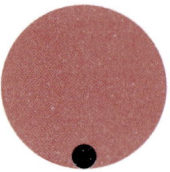

Six countries, Brazil,
Peru, Mexico,
Argentina, El
Salvador, and
Bolivia represent

70%
of violence
is committed by an
intimate or known
partner

98%
of femicides
go unprosecutes

81%
of cases

In the first weeks of lockdowns, Peru, Argetina, and **Bolivia**
saw the **largest increase** of instances of **violence.**

3/20
Argentina announces
a national quarantine.
Domestic violence
calls rise 120%

3/28
Bolivia registers
**158 cases of domestic
violence** in its first
week of quarantine

3/15
Peru announces a national
quarantine, **restricting the
movement of women** to
Tuesdays, Thursdays, and
Saturdays

3/21
Bolivia announces a national
quarantine.

3/31
The Peruvian Ministry for
women receives **600 calls**
and **registered 168 cases**
of violence against
women.

The effects of **Quarantines** and work restrictions

Isolate women
at home

decrease access
to **social justice**

and heighten the risk of
gender-based violence
and **femicide.**

By Alexander Borushek and Beatriz Nice
Data provided by the UN Organization for women and CEPAL

Figure 2.3: Shadow pandemic

CONCLUSION

The shadow or silent pandemic as gender-based violence is known which includes domestic violence has unfortunately reached enormous proportions and according to estimates by UN women is 243 million women have been subjected to gender-based violence which includes domestic violence since the past 12 months. Unfortunately, COVID crisis has stretched the health care systems globally to the breaking point and has reduced the available resources to address the shadow pandemic. The way forward that if we as a global community want to promote health and well-being for all in social and recovery efforts and strengthen our existing health care systems and delivery especially for women and girls they need to be included in the front and center of decision making and response.

REFERENCES

1. Center for Global Development (2020). Pandemics and Violence Against Women and Children. Working Paper 528 Accessed October 4 https://www.cgdev.org/sites/default/files/pandemics-and-vawg-april2.pdf

2. UN Women. 2020. UN Secretary-General's Policy Brief: The Impact Of COVID-19 On Women |Digital Library: Publications. [online]. Accessed October 4 Available at: https://www.unwomen.org/en/digital-library/publications/2020/04/policy-brief-the-impact-of-covid-19-on-women.

3. United Nations Population Fund (2018) Recovering from the Ebola Virus Disease: Rapid Assessment of Pregnant Adolescent Girls in Sierra Leone. Accessed October 4 https://sierraleone.unfpa.org/en/publications/recovering-ebola-virus-disease-rapid-assessment-pregnant-adolescent-girls-sierra-leone.

4. Data 2 X Buvinic M, Noe L, Swanson E. Tracking the gender Impact of COVID-19 https://data2x.org/tracking-the-gender-impact-of-covid-19/. Accessed October 4.

3

European Online Training Platform on Domestic Violence— Improving Frontline Responses to Domestic Violence and Sexual Assault

Bettina Pfleiderer, Paulina Juszczyk

Abstract

Health professionals are often the first point of contact for victims of domestic violence and thus play a major role in the detection and intervention of domestic violence. Interviews with professionals from the medical sector within the EU IMPRODOVA research project (www.improdova.eu) indicated that they are not sufficiently trained in domestic violence and that they are not aware of their role as frontline responders in cases of domestic violence. It also became clear that interagency collaboration was lacking. IMPRODOVA designed therefore training formats and materials not only for the health sector but also for the police and the social sector to improve frontline responders' competencies to prevent, investigate and mitigate domestic violence. In this article, we are presenting the IMPRODOVA online training platform (www.training.improdova.eu) with a focus on the medical sector.

The IMPRODOVA Project and its Methodology

The IMPRODOVA project (https://www.improdova.eu)—improving frontline responses to high impact domestic violence—is a search and innovation project funded by the European Union. It involves a group of experienced researchers and practitioners from eight European countries: Austria, Finland, France, Germany, Hungary, Portugal, Slovenia, and UK (Scotland) working together to provide solutions for an integrated response to high impact domestic violence (HIDV), based on comprehensive empirical research of how police, medical and social work professionals respond to domestic violence in European countries. IMPRODOVA's operational definition of high impact domestic violence (HIDV) is serious violence within the family, against children, spouses and elderly family members. Seriousness can be intensity, duration and consequences of violence.

IMPRODOVA started in May 2018 with a duration of 36 months. Due to the current COVID-19 situation, the project will be extended by four months. In **phase 1**, IMPRODOVA started with the analysis of policy implementation, legislation, data, risk assessment, case documentation, cooperation, and trainings, including the status quo of the medical profession related to domestic violence (DV). In **phase 2**, 296 interviews with different frontline responders from the police, the health sector, and the social sector in eight European countries were conducted to investigate frontline responder practices with a special emphasis on interagency cooperation to assess the extent to which standards are converted into practice and the actors being involved in multi-professional approaches to tackle DV. In **phase 3**, the project developed tool kits addressing for example risk assessment practices and a training platform with various training materials was designed to improve a multi-agency collaboration. All those tools and the training platform are currently being evaluated, and the feedback given will be used to further optimize them to the need of the practitioners being part of DV frontline response. Figure 3.1 summarizes the timeline of the project.

In theory, we know very well how to prevent, detect and mitigate domestic violence. However, in daily practice these recommendations and guidelines are not always implemented. Across Europe, there are examples of good practices from which we can learn. For instance, in some countries (e.g. Germany) programmes exist that promote the involvement of the medical profession in domestic violence fighting networks (e.g.https://training.improdova.eu/en/training-modules-for-the-social-sector/module-7-principles-of-interorganisational-cooperation-and-risk-assessment-in-cases-of-domestic-violence-in-multi-professional-eams/2/) and have received good outcomes. This best practice examples have been collated by the IMPRODOVA consortium and are shared via the training platform.

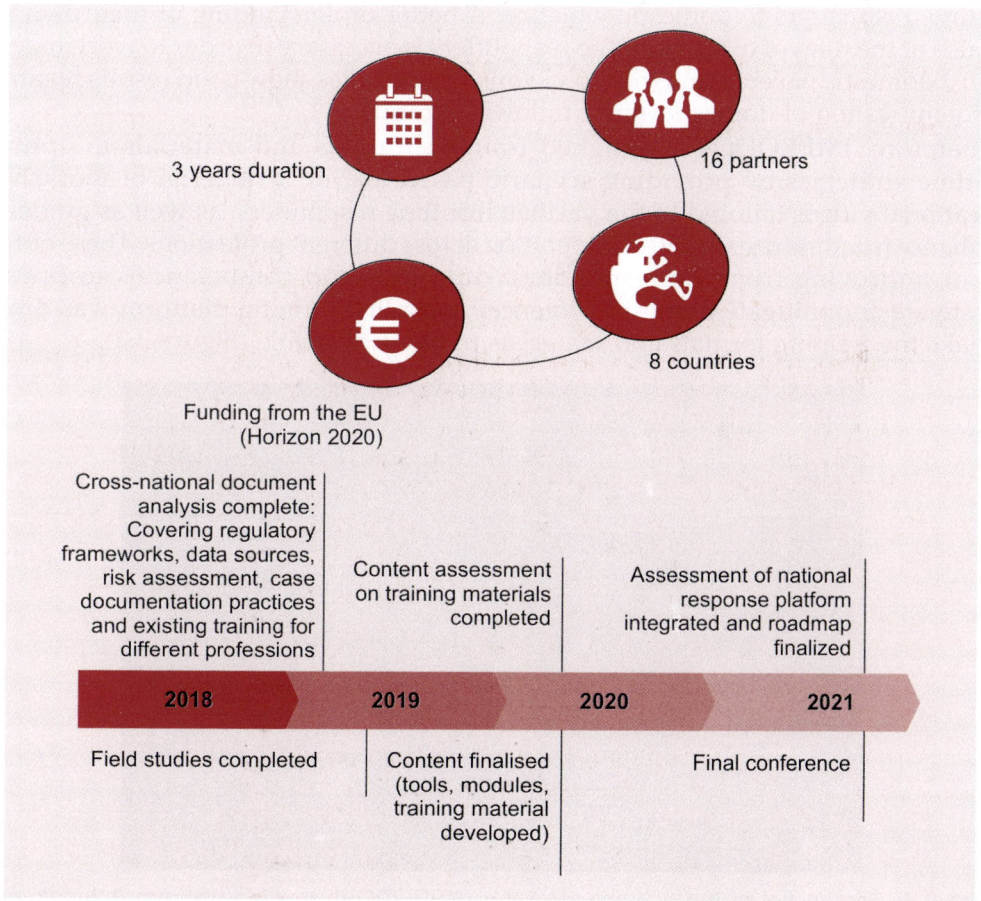

Figure 3.1: Timeline of the IMPRODOVA project

Why the Health Sector Needs Training on Domestic Violence?

Domestic violence can lead to short- and long-term health consequences, prompting victims of domestic violence to seek help from the medical profession. For this reason, health professionals are often the first point of contact for victims of domestic violence and thus play a major role in the detection and intervention of domestic violence. General practitioners, emergency physicians, emergency paramedics, gynecologists, midwives and nurses as well as dentists[1] are the health professionals who most frequently encounter victims of domestic violence and thereby among those who first hear about an incident or perceive indicators or symptoms of domestic violence. The medical profession is not only considered by the Istanbul Convention;[2] (Article 18 (114); Article 20 (127); Article 22 (132); Article 25 (141)) to be an important stakeholder, but its role is also highlighted by numerous authors in research studies.[3–5]

However, based on the interviews with health professionals in the IMPRODOVA countries, it has become apparent that they are not sufficiently trained in domestic violence. Knowledge about domestic violence, symptoms and red flags are often not part of the mandatory curriculum for physicians or at medical school for medical students in most European countries. Therefore, many health professionals are not aware of the important role they play in the network. They see their role primarily in taking care of the medical needs of their patients and rarely consider themselves as frontline responders to domestic violence. A better understanding of their own role, but also of the roles of other frontline responders is necessary in order to work together against domestic violence and to help victims. First studies show good results regarding the identification of domestic abuse following trainings.[6]

Therefore, IMPRODOVA designed training formats and materials to optimize frontline strategies by providing scenario-based learning, material of workshops, educational videos tailored to the various frontline responders, as well as guidelines to enhance frontline responders' cooperation across different professions. These outputs aim at improving frontline responders' capacities and competencies to prevent, investigate and mitigate domestic violence. An online training platform was drafted to make the training formats and materials publicly available (Figure 3.2).

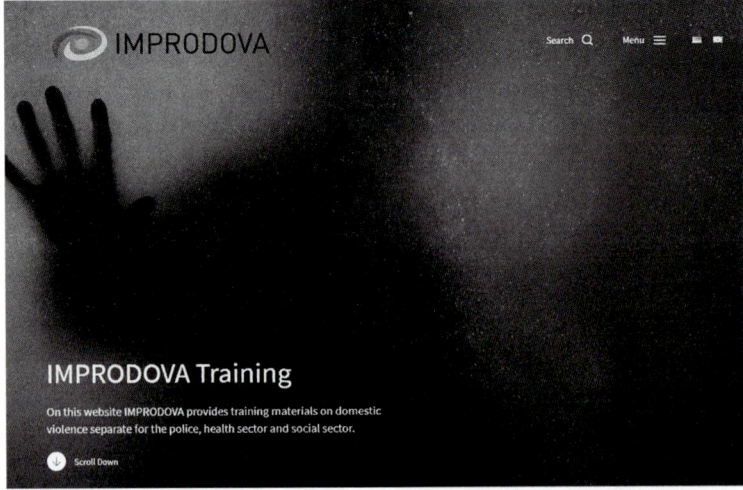

Figure 3.2: Screenshot of the homepage of the IMPRODOVA training platform (https://training.improdova.eu/)

Training Modules on Domestic Violence or Why Knowledge is Power

The IMPRODOVA training platform addresses three main frontline responder groups: The police, the health sector and professionals from NGOs and the social sector. It is modular and consists of seven modules for each frontline responder group, which are thematically the same, but with adapted content to the sector (Figure 3.3). **Module 1 (forms and dynamics of domestic violence)** aims at gaining a better understanding of domestic violence and its forms and consequences. Knowledge is transmitted about the specific contexts and the impact of domestic abuse that can be a helpful step in understanding the individual needs of victims. The objective of **Module 2 (indicators of domestic violence)** is to become familiar with the various indicators for domestic violence, their related risks and to be sensitised to them. As one of the first points of contact, health professionals have the opportunity to identify victims of domestic violence at a relatively early stage and ensure that victims receive the individual support they need quickly. **Module 3 (communication in cases of domestic violence)** presents the different ways of asking about domestic violence in situations where a frontline responder suspects the presence of domestic violence. Furthermore, first steps after the disclosure of domestic violence are presented. Especially, medical staff can stay in contact with victims afterwards and follow-up their situation. **Module 4 for the police (police investigation and legal proceedings)** presents the most important aspects to be considered in police investigations and subsequent legal proceedings after the disclosure of domestic violence. **Module 4 for the health sector (medical assessment and securing of evidence)** presents the most important aspects to be considered after the disclosure of domestic violence and how to document domestic violence injuries for legal trials. It explains in particular how the securing of evidence by a physician can be done in such way that it can be used as evidence in court. **Module 4 for the social sector (support services of the social sector)** presents the help offered by social services after the disclosure of domestic violence. Different contact points are introduced to the reader. **Module 5 (risk assessment and safety planning)** presents why risk assessment is such an important step when tackling domestic violence and what needs to be considered when assessing the risk of victims of domestic violence and what steps are necessary to improve the safety of victims. Knowing these facts, health professionals could intervene long before victims would make the decision to leave the perpetrator or report the incident to the police. **Module 6 (international standards and legal frameworks in Europe)** introduces the international framework in which the work of frontline responders takes place and also presents country-specific regulations in order to gain an impression of how other European countries tackle

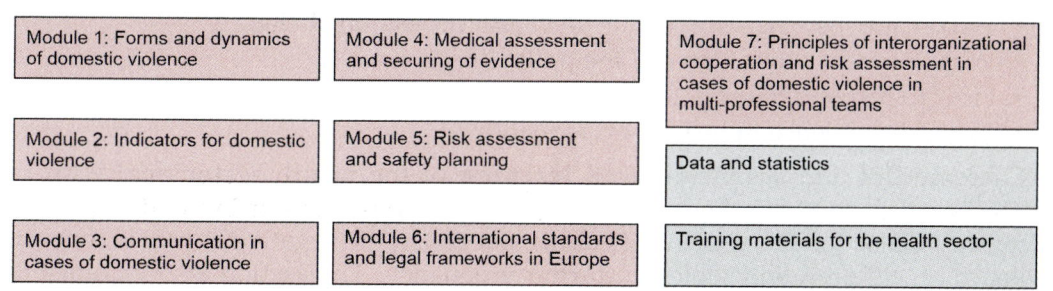

Figure 3.3: Training modules being included in the IMPRODOVA training platform on domestic violence for the health sector

domestic violence. The aim of **Module 7 (principles of interorganizational cooperation and risk assessment in cases of domestic violence in multi-professional teams)** is to understand how frontline responders work and why cooperation in multi-professional teams is most successful in tackling domestic violence.

The Recurring Problem of Limited Time Resources

15 minutes sections are implemented for the police, the health sector and the social sector, where the most important information for the three frontline responder groups is summarized hereby considering the limited time resources of practitioners. Because of the tight schedule and the shortage of human resources, speaking with victims about domestic violence is usually considered as almost impossible by physicians. The aim of this tailored section for the medical sector **"Domestic violence in the health sector in 15 minutes"** is to support practitioners in identifying patients and their children who have been victims of domestic violence and to respond to them appropriately in a very short time. It gives an overview of possible indicators for domestic violence and its physical and psychological consequences. Beyond that, it includes guidelines for patient care and some legal information.

The Necessary Tools

In addition to the seven modules and 15 minutes sections, information regarding **data and statistics** is presented for all frontline responder groups in a separate section. The section includes information about victimization surveys and police data in the EU as those sources have produced most reliable and extensive data available. Additionally, recommendations on good data harmonization and consolidation that should be regarded, are summarized.

 Training videos, case studies and **scenario-based learning, knowledge assessments**, and downloadable **factsheets** and **presentations**, as well as an exemplary **workshop concept** for the health sector, that can be adapted by trainers, can be found in the various modules or can be selected separately from the teaching materials. The training videos were produced on the following topics:

- Domestic violence in times of disasters.
- The UN and their role in combating violence against women.
- Why is cooperation in cases of domestic violence important?
- Who are the perpetrators of domestic violence?
- Who are the victims of domestic violence?
- What happens when you contact a victim protection shelter?
- What happens when you call the police?
- How to respond to a disclosure?
- Domestic violence in health services.

 Case studies and **scenario-based learning** of the health sector deal with the disclosure of domestic violence to the primary care physician or in medical practice, domestic violence affecting mental health, elder abuse, the negative impact of domestic violence on children and violence during pregnancy. The section also includes the IMPRODOVA risk assessment integration module that explains the whole risk assessment procedure for a specific case (Figure 3.4).

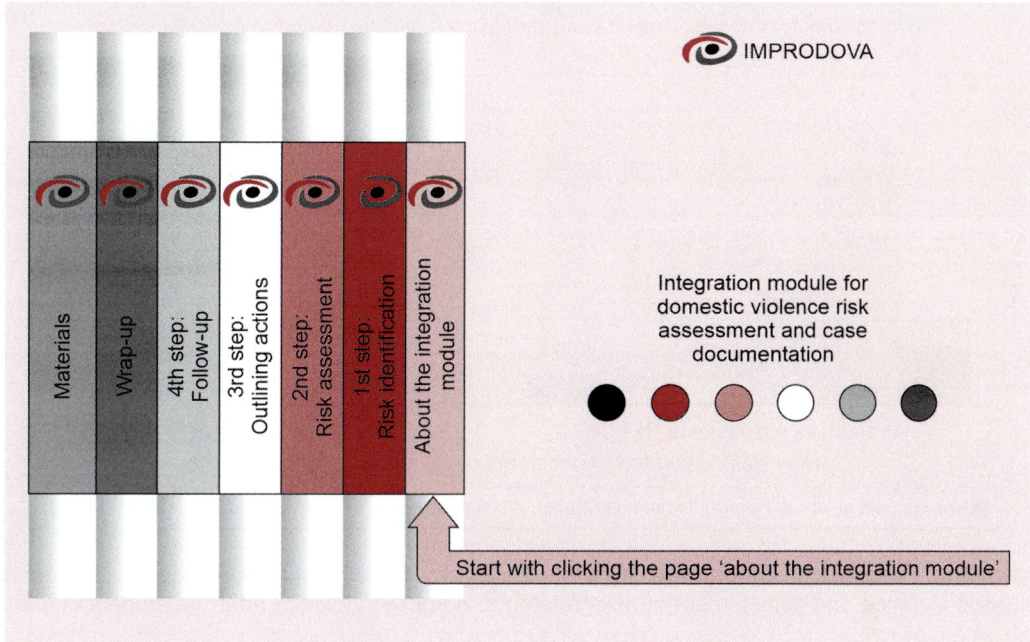

Figure 3.4: Screenshot of the integration module for domestic violence risk assessment and case documentation on the platform. Online link: https://training.improdova.eu/wp-content/uploads/2020/08/Improdova_Risk_Assessment_Integration_Module_Final.pptx

The Missing Pieces

As mentioned before, the IMPRODOVA training platform presents an overview of domestic violence on the EU level and corresponding policies, but does not necessarily reflect national or local contexts. Therefore, as a best practice model for a national version of the international training platform a German IMPRODOVA training platform was developed (https://training.improdova.eu/de/). The whole IMPRODOVA training platform and related materials were translated into German and adapted to the German context.

Assessment of the IMPRODOVA Training Platform or Getting Better and Better

The assessment of the IMPRODOVA training platform serves to further optimize the training materials offered. Both the English and the German training platforms are currently being evaluated. An elective student course has been developed (28 hr) and was held already twice—due to the Corona Pandemic online—on the topic "Domestic violence in an International Context" at the medical faculty in Münster. The course was based on the German training platform. First feedback results revealed that the training platform, including its teaching materials, has resulted in a significant learning and competence progress of the students in all subject areas (Figures 3.5 and 3.6). Also, the students' interest in regional cooperation with other frontline responders, which was lower as compared to other topics prior to the student class, increased after the class. Our students were particularly interested in the communication with victims in cases of domestic violence and in the case studies offered on the training platform.

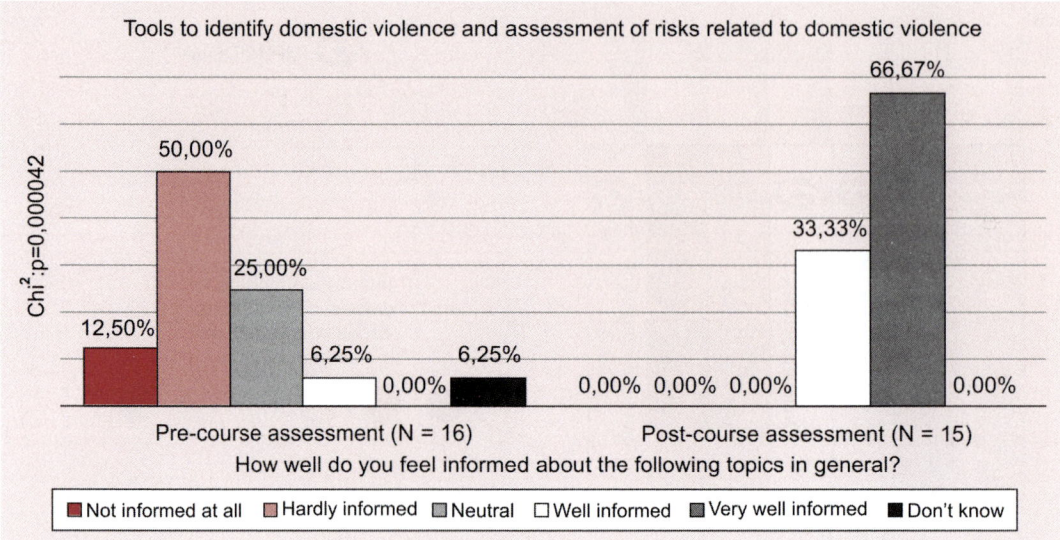

Figure 3.5: Feedback of students indicated that they felt much better informed about tools to identify domestic violence and assessment of risks related to domestic violence after the student course

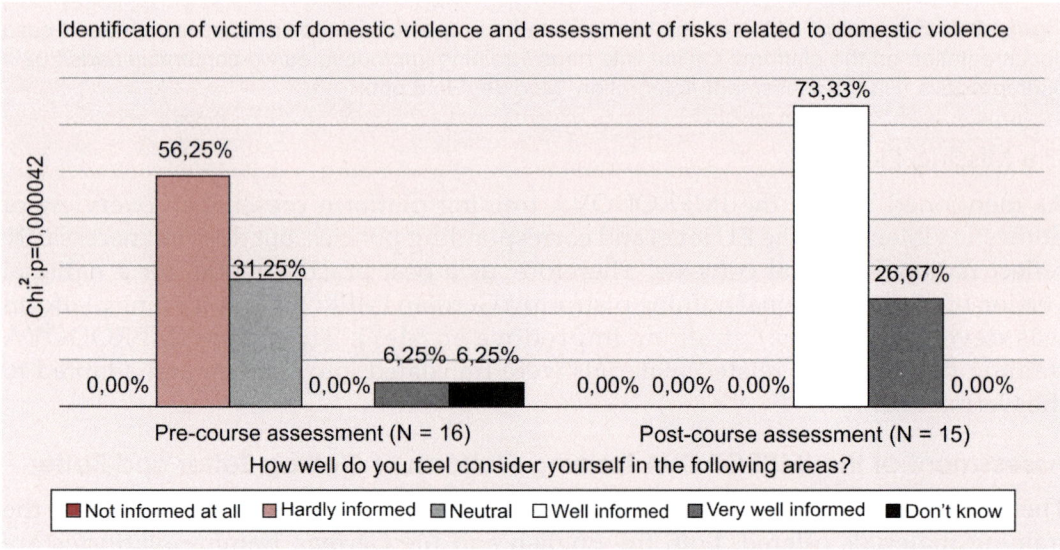

Figure 3.6: Feedback of students showed they felt more competent about the identification of victims of domestic violence and assessment of risks related to domestic violence after the student course

The feedback also indicated that there are still some gaps in the content of the platform that need to be filled. For this reason, work is already underway on supplementary content on domestic violence in the media, domestic violence in times of COVID-19 and information tailored to school teachers.

Acknowledgement

This project has received funding from the European Union's Horizon 2020 research and innovation programme under grant agreement No. 787054. This article reflects only the authors' view and the European Commission is not responsible for any use that may be made of the information it contains.

REFERENCES

1. Ellis TW, Brownstein S, Beitchman K, Lifshitz J. Restoring More than Smiles in Broken Homes: Dental and Oral Biomarkers of Brain Injury in Domestic Violence. J Aggress Maltreat Trauma [Internet]. 2019 Apr [cited 2020 Dec 9];28(7):838-847. Available from: https://doi.org/10.1080/10926771.2019.1595803.

2. Council of Europe. Convention on preventing and combating violence against women and domestic violence. Council of Europe Treaty Series-No. 210. 2011 [cited 2020 Nov 27]. Available from: www.coe.int/conventionviolence.

3. Alsaedi JA, Elbarrany WG, Al Majnon WA, Al-Namankany AA. Barriers that Impede Primary Health Care Physicians from Screening Women for Domestic Violence at Makkah ALmukarramah City. Egypt J Hosp Med [Internet]. 2017 Oct [cited 2020 Dec 9];69(8):3058–3065. Available from: https://doi.org/10.12816/0042856.

4. Jenner SC, Etzold SS, Oesterhelweg L, Stickel A, Kurmeyer C, Reinemann D, Oertelt-Prigione S. Barriers to active inquiry about intimate partner violence among German physicians participating in a mandatory training. J Fam Violence [Internet]. 2015 Jul [cited 2020 Dec 9];31(1):109-117. Available from: https://doi.org/10.1007/s10896-015-9754-2.

5. Piterman L, Komesaroff PA, Piterman H, Jones KJ. Domestic violence: it is time for the medical profession to play its part. Intern Med J [Internet]. 2015 May 8 [cited 2020 Dec 9];45(5):471-473. Available from: https://doi.org/10.1111/imj.12738.

6. Edwardsen EA, Horwitz SH, Pless NA, le Roux HD, Fiscella KA. Improving identification and management of partner violence: examining the process of academic detailing: a qualitative study. BMC Med Educ [Internet]. 2011 Jun [cited 2020 Dec 9];11(36). Available from: https://doi.org/10.1186/1472-6920-11-36.

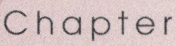

Chapter

4

WWWCON—The Way Forward

Meera Agnihotri

A new journey was started with WWW Foundation (Women Health Wellness for Women Empowerment) in collaboration with ARTIST (Asian Research and Training Institute for Skill Transfer) and IHW Council (Integrated Health and Wellbeing Council), details of which are discussed here as the way forward to help survivors.

Background

Prof Meera Agnihotri, Chief Patron, Kanpur ObGy Society (KOGS) received the most prestigious Women Empowerment National Award at AICOG (All India Conference of Obstetrics and Gynaecology) on 21st Jan 2018 at Bhubaneshwar, Odisha. There after she was bestowed with the honor to organize WWWCON International Conference, FOGSI (Women Health and Wellness for Woman Empowerment) as Organizing Chairperson. We were really blessed that for the first time in the history of FOGSI Hon'ble President of India Shri Ramnath Kovind Ji had agreed to inaugurate this conference. In this event, women's health issues from womb to tomb were discussed. Health sanitation, hygiene, medical, social, spiritual all aspects were covered by Stalwarts, including 200 national and international faculty. Representatives of state including UP ministers and Mayor of Kanpur participated in the Public Forum held on the issue of prevention of violence against women.

Mission and Message of Dr Meera Agnihotri (Founder)

Being Medical Doctor   — Treating Patience is my Profession
Being Medical Teacher — Teaching is my duty and Privilege
                                Women Empowerment is my Passion

Being inspired by recognition of my work for Women Empowerment activities we have transformed WWWCON blessed by President of India and Union Health Minister into WWW Foundation. With the same aims and objectives to empower our women and transform the status of females in our country.

The issue of **Women Empowerment** is a **Global Concern and one of the prime agendas** of WHO (World Health Organization) and it is one of the greatest concerns of our country. The Global scenario of women health wellness is well-known; it needs a

U-turn to empower our women with the different health agendas including **medical health, maternal diet and nutrition, empowering women the motherhood, spiritual evolution, making them disease free, vaccination against preventable diseases, improving reproductive health of women and many more.**

In India, although a number of policies are provided **by central and state governments** and many more are in pipeline will be met, yet women in our country are still looked upon as 2nd grade in the man dominated (patriarchal society).

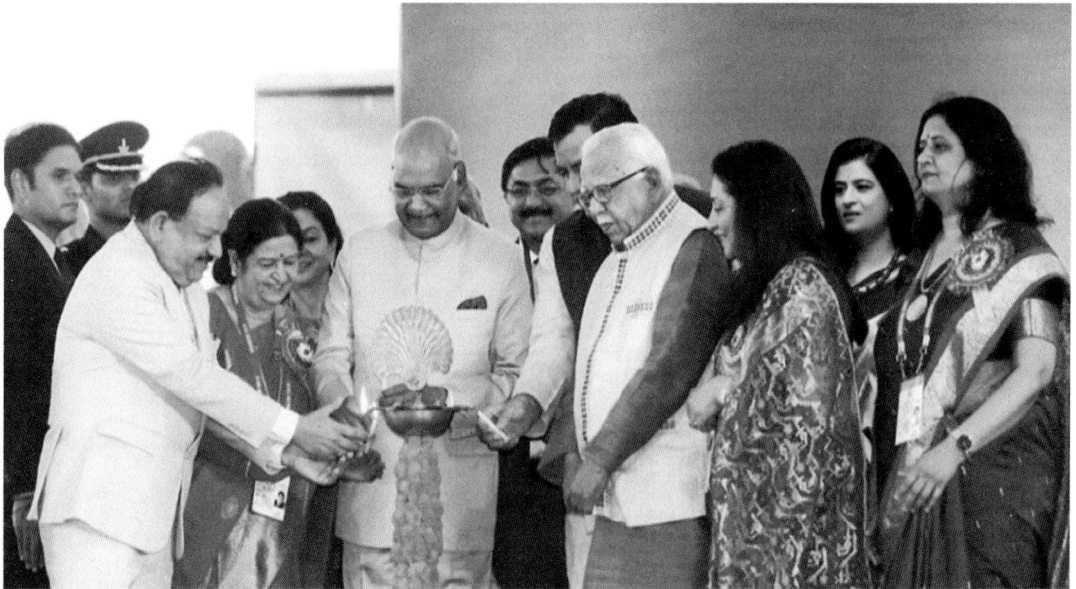

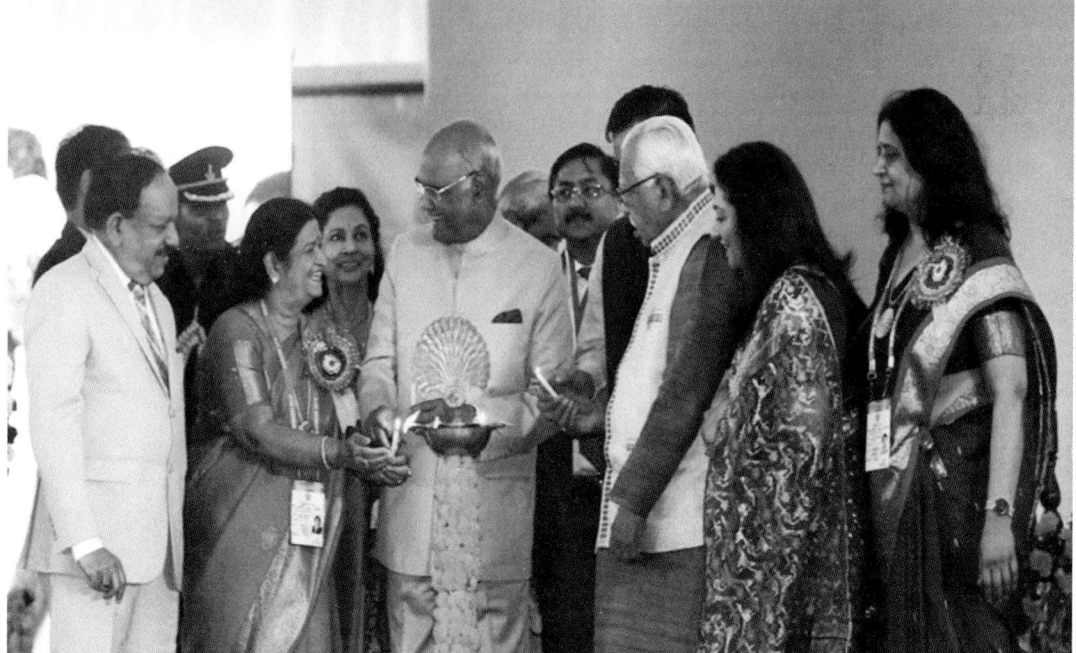

Figure 4.1: WWWCON 2018 Inauguration by Hon President of India

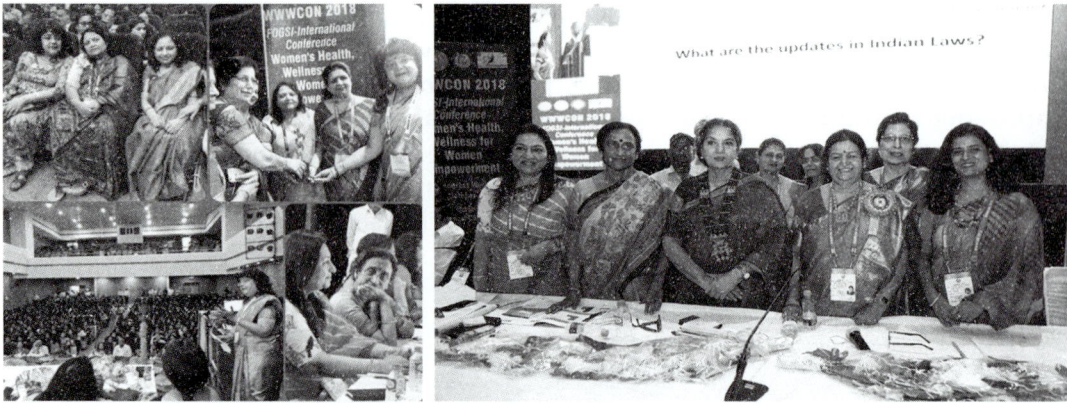

Figure 4.2: WWWCON 2018 Panel discussion with FOGSI Stalwarts, Politicians and Media

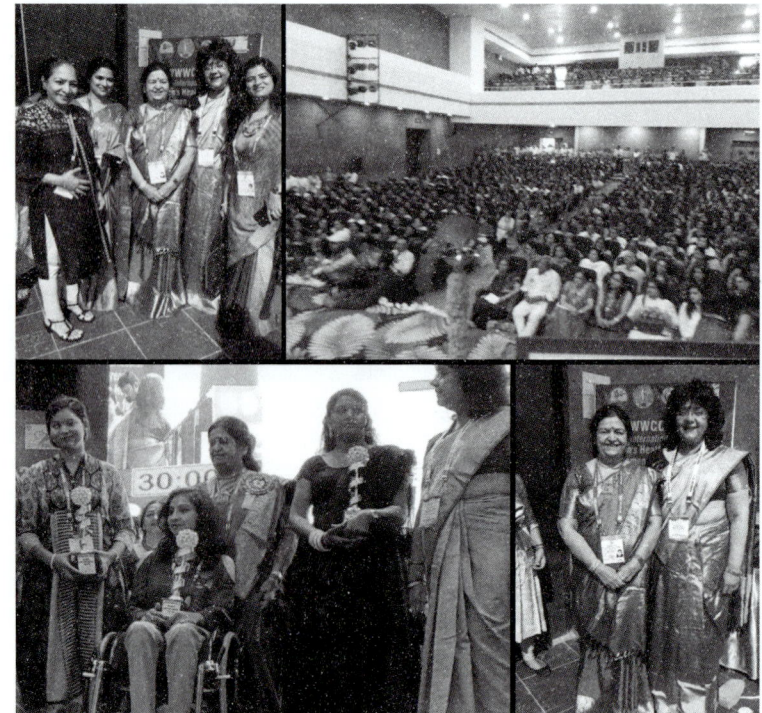

Figure 4.3: WWWCON Public Forum Dr Meera Agnihotri and Dr Reena Wani

Six "S" are Basically Needed to Empower the Women

Shiksha = Education
Swasthya = Health
Swavlamban = Self Reliance
Samajik Nyay = Justice
Samvedan = Sensitivity
Samta = Equality

Social Obstetrics is one of the most important 7th tools Empowering Women.

It can change the basic concept of all the **SIX "S" needed to empower women**. This book covers **each and every aspect right from "Womb-to-tomb"**. The journey of humanity in womb starts right from two different cells; ovum from mother and sperm from father, zygote implanting *in utero* and the transformation into a complete human being in short span of nine months is most fascination. Fetus is our second patient who is privileged with "Right of unborn child". It is entirely the jurisdiction of obstetricians to **protect the unborn legally, medically, socially, and spiritually**.

Therefore, the face of antenatal care has undergone revolutionary change and a paradigm shift in the last couple of decades with the advent of fetal medicine. Obstetrics has now diversified into a dual care pathway addressing the needs of mother and the fetus as two different patients rather than common entity. It needs further Empowering Mother.

FOGSI focus was released at WWWCON: In this book efforts are made to include and discuss the latest **concept in health issues related to women** in an attempt to empower than as it carries all the issues of **obstetrics and gynecology including social obstetrics. This received best Publication Award in AICOG, Lucknow 2020.**

Plans for Implementation

Initially 4 geographical zones (N, S, E, W) were identified but the need to have activities in each state was felt to be pressing hence decision has been taken to have a coordinator in each state to take forward the activities for Women Empowerment.

She will restart a new life, new mission, new commitment
She needs our support in addition to government support

Laws and Vaw

Domestic Violence Act, 2005

Mandakini Megh, Preeti Deshpande

Introduction

Domestic violence is a major issue in all strata of Indian society till today. Contrary to the belief, domestic violence is also seen in higher socio-economic classes but reporting is poor to avoid publicity and media coverage.

United Nations has organized four world conferences on women over the decades. The 1995 Fourth World Conference on Women in Beijing marked a significant turning point for the global agenda for gender equality. The Beijing Declaration and Platform for Action was adopted unanimously in 189 countries. It has an agenda for women's empowerment and considered the key global document on gender equality. It sets strategic objectives and actions for the advancement of women in critical areas of concern such as women and poverty, training of women, health, violence against women, the girl child, human rights and media issues related to women.

From time to time various Acts have been passed for the cause of women in India.

- The Dowry Prohibition Act, 1961
- The Equal Remuneration Act, 1976
- The Child Marriage Restrain Act, 1976
- The Medical Termination of Pregnancy Act, 1971
- The National Commission for Women Act, 1990
- The Protection of Human Rights Act, 1993
- Protection of Women from Domestic Violence Act, 2005[1]
- Sexual Harassment at Workplace (Prevention, Prohibition and Redressal) Act, 2013.

In 2020, Domestic violence against women remained a prime concern for the Ministry of Women and Child Development with over 5,000 complaints received in the year. The National Commission for Women (NCW) was flooded with complaints for domestic violence in March as the lockdown was imposed and it forced women to remain confined at home with their abusers. Economic insecurity, financial instability and isolation triggered a rise in domestic violence. It also reduced their chance to access help. Also protection officers and police could not reach out to their home to help. NCW launched a new 'WhatsApp helpline number' for emergency response.[2]

We need to fight against domestic violence as a society. Let us see in detail the provisions of the Protection of Women Against Domestic Violence Act, 2005.

Patterns of Violence

Married women are more likely to experience physical and sexual violence by husbands (Figure 5.1). Nearly 36% of married women have experienced some form of physical or sexual violence by their husband. For never married women, the most common perpetrators include mothers or step-mothers, fathers or step-fathers, sisters or brothers and teachers.[3]

Patterns of Physical Violence

- Women's experience of physical violence increases with age from 17% at 15–19 years to 35% at 40–49 years.
- Physical violence is more in rural areas (32%) than in urban areas (25%).
- Women's experience of physical violence declines sharply with education (from 41% in those with no schooling to 17% in women with 12 or more years of schooling).

Patterns of Sexual Violence

- Women's experience of sexual violence increases with age from 3% at 15–19 years to 5% at 20–24 years.
- Single or divorced women experience more sexual violence (13%).
- Sexual violence is also higher in rural areas (36% *vs* 28%).

Protection of Women Against Domestic Violence Act (PWDVA), 2005[1] (Table 5.1)

Domestic violence is recognized as a criminal offence under IPC 498A. After enactment of the Protection of Women from Domestic Violence Act, 2005 additional protection was given to victims of domestic violence. Cases under Domestic Violence Act go to the criminal court. Any case of domestic violence in areas with a population of 10 lakhs or more such as Mumbai district would first go to a Metropolitan Magistrate. For smaller towns the cases would go to an equivalent First Class Judicial Magistrate. In case the aggrieved person wants to go to a higher court, she would need to go to a Sessions Court and subsequently the High Court.

Main Features of the Act

The definition of an 'aggrieved person' is equally wide and covers not just the wife but a woman who is the sexual partner of the male irrespective of whether she is his legal wife or not. The daughter, mother, sister, child (male or female), widowed relative, in fact, any woman residing in the household who is related in some way to the respondent, is also covered by the Act.

The respondent under the definition given in the Act is "any male, adult person who is, or has been, in a domestic relationship with the aggrieved person" but so that his mother, sister and other relatives do not go scot free, the case can also be filed against relatives of the husband or male partner.

The information regarding an Act or Acts of domestic violence does not necessarily have to be lodged by the aggrieved party but by "any person who has reason to believe that" such an Act has been or is being committed. This means that neighbours, social workers, relatives, etc. can all take initiative on behalf of the victim.

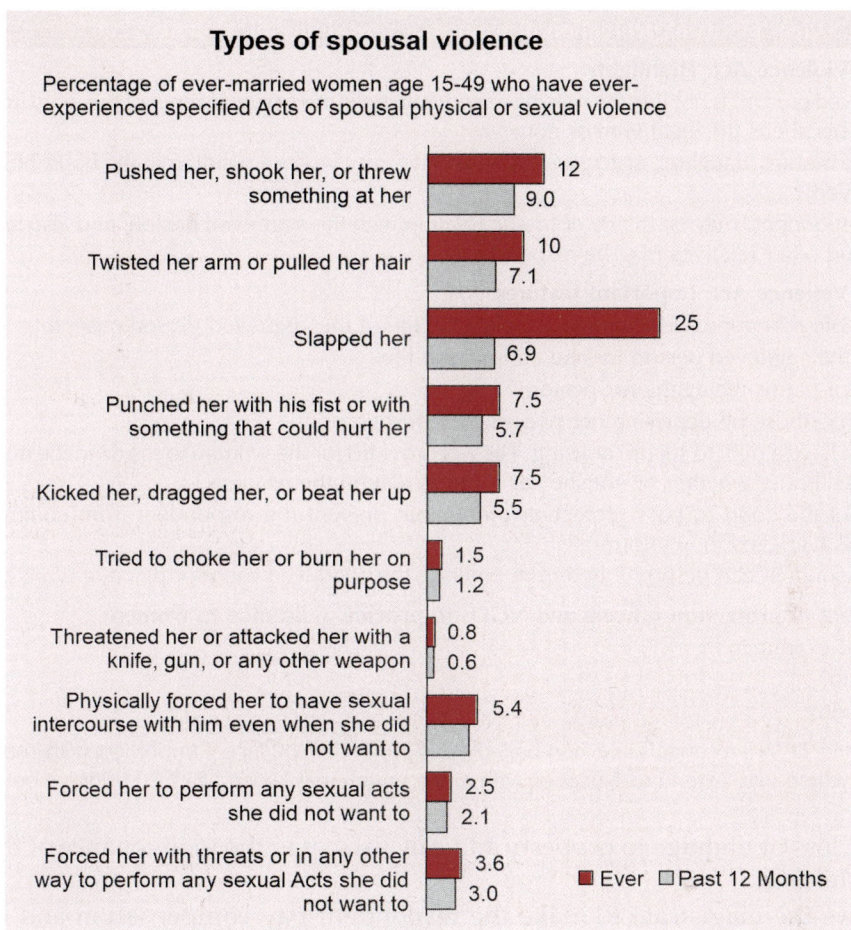

Types of spousal violence

Percentage of ever-married women age 15-49 who have ever-experienced specified Acts of spousal physical or sexual violence

Pushed her, shook her, or threw something at her — 12 / 9.0

Twisted her arm or pulled her hair — 10 / 7.1

Slapped her — 25 / 6.9

Punched her with his fist or with something that could hurt her — 7.5 / 5.7

Kicked her, dragged her, or beat her up — 7.5 / 5.5

Tried to choke her or burn her on purpose — 1.5 / 1.2

Threatened her or attacked her with a knife, gun, or any other weapon — 0.8 / 0.6

Physically forced her to have sexual intercourse with him even when she did not want to — 5.4

Forced her to perform any sexual acts she did not want to — 2.5 / 2.1

Forced her with threats or in any other way to perform any sexual Acts she did not want to — 3.6 / 3.0

■ Ever ☐ Past 12 Months

Figure 5.1: Forms of spousal violence experienced by ever-married women in percentage[3]

This fear of being driven out of the house effectively silenced many women and made them silent sufferers. The court, by this Act, can now order that she not only reside in the same house but that a part of the house can even be allotted to her for her personal use even if she has no legal claim or share in the property.

It allows the magistrate to protect the woman from Acts of violence or even "Acts that are likely to take place" in the future and can prohibit the respondent from dispossessing the aggrieved person or in any other manner disturbing her possessions, entering the aggrieved person's place of work or, if the aggrieved person is a child, the school.

The respondent can also be restrained from attempting to communicate in any form, whatsoever, with the aggrieved person, including personal, oral, written, electronic or telephonic contact. The respondent can even be prohibited from entering the room/area of the house that is allotted to her by the court.

The Act allows magistrates to impose monetary relief and monthly payments of maintenance. The respondent can also be made to meet the expenses incurred and losses suffered by the aggrieved person and expenses of any child of the aggrieved person as a result of domestic violence and can also cover loss of earnings, medical

Table 5.1: Salient points of protection of women against domestic violence, 2005

Domestic Violence Act: Highlights

1. 'Aggrieved person' is not just the wife by a woman who is the sexual partner of the male irrespective of whether she is the legal wife or not
2. Also the mother, daughter, sister, widowed relative, any woman residing in the household may be "aggrieved"
3. The "respondent" may be in any domestic relation with the aggrieved person, and also his mother, sister and other relatives may be respondents.

Domestic Violence Act: Important features

1. Applicable if he repeated assaults or makes the life of the aggrieved person miserable
2. Forces the aggrieved person to lead an immoral life
3. Injures or harms the aggrieved person
4. Economic abuse by depriving her of economic resources
5. Women have a right to secure housing. The Act provides for the woman to reside in the matrimonial or shared house whether or not she has rights to stay in the property
6. Power of the court to pass protection orders that prevent the respondent from communicating with the aggrieved in any form
7. The respondent can be prohibited from entering the aggrieved room or place of work or school.

Appointment of protection officers and NGOs to provide assistance to women

1. Medical examination
2. Legal aid
3. Safe shelter

Offence under DVA is a congnisable, non-bailable and punishable offence. Punishment with imprisonment for a term which may extend to 1 year or with a fine which may extend to ₹ 20,000/- or both.

expenses, loss or damage to property and can also cover the maintenance of the victim and her children.

It allows the magistrate to make the respondent pay compensation and damages for injuries including mental torture and emotional distress caused by Acts of domestic violence. It gives a penalty up to one year imprisonment and/or a fine up to ₹ 20,000/- for the offence. The offence is also considered cognizable and non-bailable.

It goes even further and says that "under the sole testimony of the aggrieved person, the court may conclude that an offence has been committed by the accused".

The Act also ensures speedy justice as the court has to start proceedings and have the first hearing within 3 days of the complaint being filed in court and every case must be disposed of within a period of sixty days of the first hearing.

It makes provisions for the state to provide for protection officers and the whole machinery by which to implement the Act. It is the role of protection officers to assist the magistrate in the discharge of his functions. They are supposed to make the domestic incident report. They are supposed to ensure that legal aid is provided to the aggrieved person. They are to maintain a list of service providers, shelter homes and medical facilities. Their role is also to ascertain that the aggrieved person gets monetary relief.

The Act also provides for the penalty for not discharging duty of protection officer.

The Acts enunciate the certain duties of central and state governments to make wide publicity and arrange training programs for the police officers.

The Act also provides for the assistance of welfare experts if found necessary by the magistrate.

The Act recommends service providers to facilitate the processes. Any voluntary association registered under the Societies Registration Act, 1860 or a company registered under the Companies Act, 1956 or any other law in force with the objective of protecting the rights of women shall register itself as a service provider. A service provider can record the domestic incidence report in prescribed form if the aggrieved person desires and forward a copy to the protection officer or magistrate. The service provider can get the aggrieved person medically examined and forward the medical report to the protection officer and police station. The service provider can ensure shelter is provided to the aggrieved person if she so desires. No legal suit can lie against the service provider who is deemed to be acting in good faith to prevent domestic violence.

Loopholes in the Present System, Unclarified Responsibility and Insufficient Official Resource

In practice duty of each role such as the protection officers and service providers still seems ambiguous.

Lack of Training of Police Officers

There is a lack of training of police officers and magistrates regarding the Act's requirements and its purpose, as well as a lack of sensitivity training towards the issue of domestic violence. This lack of training has led to the re-victimisation of women within the justice system, either through police's non-response to calls for help, sending women back home to their abusers by branding their victimisation as mere domestic disputes, or magistrates allowing for numerous hearings of cases, prolonging the court process and forcing victims to come to court to face their trauma time and again.

Dual System: Family Court and Criminal Court

There are mainly two legal approaches for women, who had suffered domestic violence, one is filing for divorce through family court, and the other is filing application to magistrate according to Domestic Violence Act which goes through Criminal Legal System. The dual system sometimes makes the legal proceeding more complex even tedious for them. Also, the social impression of each approach put some stress on them.

Drawbacks of the Domestic Violence Act

The Act is deeply controversial due its insistence that firstly, the person who commits domestic violence is always a male, and secondly, that on being accused, the onus is on the man to prove his innocence. Therefore, there are a lot of chances of the Act being misused by unscrupulous women.

In attempting to anticipate all possible ways to protect all aggrieved women from any sort of harm, the framers of the law have put their faith in all women being essentially honest victims.

Disparities in Implementation

There are major disparities in implementation of the law in various states. Not surprisingly, states that invested in implementation of the Act in terms of funds and personnel also reported the highest number of cases filed.

Fading Attempts of NGOs as Service Provider

Very few NGOs have registered themselves as service providers under the Act, the registered service providers as well as protection officers lack experience with domestic violence work and few protection officers are assigned in each district to handle the case load.

Failure to Mandate Criminal Penalties

Advocates and protection officers have noted additional inadequacies of the PWDVA, including the Act's failure to mandate criminal penalties for abuse along with its civil measures, its failure to explicitly provide a maximum duration of appellate hearings which delays women's grant of relief, the residency orders failure to give women substantive property rights to the shared household (only giving them the right to reside there), and a basic lack of infrastructure linking law enforcement officials, officials under the Act, and service providers together in order to best and most efficiently serve domestic violence victims.

Shaking Responsibilities

The Act has by and large affected those who have access to quality legal aid. Though the Act provides for state legal aid, the quality of services in such cases is really poor. The state has passed on all responsibility to the service providers. They have to provide medical aid to abused women, arrange for short stay homes and arrange for compensation. It becomes a burden on these providers who do not have the wherewithal.

Lack of Follow-up

Needless to say, lack of follow-up can endanger victims' safety as well as allow for corruption and inefficiency within the organizations intended to help them. In addition, a Times of India, July 19th, 2009 article reported the PWDVA's lack of retroactivity, citing the Mumbai High Court's decision to set aside an order permitting an abused woman to reside in her husband's flat since his eviction attempt occurred prior to the PWDVA's enactment in 2005.

Victims of domestic violence may hide such incidents. Fear of community reaction and lack of support, fear that no one would believe them, feeling of shame, threat from perpetrators and lack of information about negative health consequences may prevent them from coming forward. Domestic violence is known to cause physical, emotional, social and economic consequences.

A "victim" is a person who is not fully capable of comprehending the situation at hand because of the victimhood faced. The belief is that the person so victimized that she may not be in a frame of mind to make decisions independently. Victims are also in need of compassion, care, validation and support.

CONCLUSION

The enactment of Domestic Violence Act, 2005 is an answer to violation of women's human rights which may be criminally prosecuted. Though this legislation has been thoroughly prepared, lacunas will always be there leading to accused circumventing the law.

Whether or not the Act will be misused or not only time will tell.

There cannot be any perceptible change in women's status overnight. It will take at least a decade before things change. This Act provides them a safeguard and a sort of sword in their hand so that they will not be seen as a doormat. One precondition of improving the implementation of the Domestic Violence Act is to increase women's awareness of it. Also, effective trainings for the respective roles of each department involved in the implementation of the Act are necessary. To complete the system, there should be sufficient budget invested.

In social-cultural level, to bring the idea of gender equality to public is one tough mission for the government. The process of social change is obscure however the effects are obvious. Only in a more gender-equal society, women who have suffered violence could get rid of shame/self-blame and such happenings could be de-stigmatized. Celebrities like Karishma Kapoor, Yukta Mukhey, Vanshika Dhanraj, Deepshikha Nagpal have brought their cases out in the open. This will also give courage to other women to approach the judicial system. Family, school, peer groups, and media are all agencies of social change, which all together should join the cultural revolution and mental revolution to construct India into a more female-friendly society. Domestic violence concerns so many elements. Low rates of participation in education, lack of economic independence, value biases operating against them, etc. directly and indirectly resulted in the women been given the status of being the secondary gender in Indian society.

In conclusion, I would like to quote the Israeli historian and scholar of the Holocaust; "Thou shalt not be a victim, thou shalt not be a perpetrator, but above all thou shalt not be a bystander." Domestic violence is as heinous a crime as the Holocaust.

Changing perceptions of gender education, creating and supporting peer groups can help in bringing about a positive change.

REFERENCES

1. The Protection of Women from Domestic Violence Act, 2005, No. 43 of 2005.
2. http://www.newiniandexpress.com/nation/2020/dec/25/domestic-violence-remained-serious-concern-for-wcd-ministry-in-2020-2241087.html
3. National Family Health Survey-4 (NFHS-4) 2015-2016-International Institute for Population Sciences, Deonar, Mumbai 400008, Ministry of Health and Family Welfare.

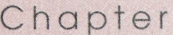

Chapter

6

Safe Workplace, a Constitutional Right of Women! Vishakha Guidelines and Beyond

Kamaxi Bhate

Vishakha sounds like a woman's name, but it connotes one of the most important milestones in the history of women's movement in India. The name of the milestone is Vishakha guidelines.

What are Vishakha guidelines? These are the guidelines issued by the Honourable Supreme Court of India, in its landmark judgement of 13th August 1997, for ensuring the safety of working women in India. The Supreme Court recognised sexual harassment at workplace as a systemic and gender-based discrimination, violating the fundamental rights of women, the right to life and liberty given by our Constitution to every citizen, as well as the principle of gender equality, which is cardinal to the Indian Constitution.

Vishakha Guidelines are a set of procedural guidelines to be followed by all establishments, public or private, in dealing with complaints about sexual harassment, until a proper and comprehensive law is enacted by Parliament for dealing with the cases of sexual harassment.

Do you know the Woman Whose Name Came to be Included in 'Vishakha Guidelines'?

Bhanwari Devi is an ordinary woman in Rajasthan, hailing from village Bhateri, which is located 55 kilometres away from capital Jaipur. She belongs to the *Kumhar* (potter) caste. Most people of the village belong to the Gurjar community of milkmen, which is higher in the caste hierarchy. Bhanwari's parents married her off at the age five or six years to a person who was only three years older.

In 1985, Bhanwari Devi became a *saathin*, a grassroots worker employed under the Women's Development Project (WDP) run by the Government of Rajasthan. *Saathins* are the last-mile change agents who work as a link between rural communities and the state government. As part of her job, she assisted the state administration in respect of issues related to land, water, literacy, health, and public distribution system (PDS). In 1987, she had to deal with a serious issue—that of an attempted rape of a woman from a neighbouring village. She showed extraordinary courage in taking up the matter, because it focused on a less-discussed social problem, she was most of the time praised by everyone in the village.

Child marriages were quite common in rural Rajasthan those days, even though they were proscribed by law. WDP tasked *saathins* with creating awareness among villagers against the age-old custom of child marriages. Bhanwari Devi took up this task with great enthusiasm, along with *prachetas* (campaigners) of the District Women's Development Agency (DWDA). The campaign was largely ignored by the villagers and faced disapproval from local leaders, including the village *pradhan* or headman.

In 1992, Bhanwari Devi came across a case of child marriage in which one Ram Karan Gurjar had planned to marry off his nine-month-old daughter. Bhanwari Devi tried to persuade the Gurjar family against carrying out the wedding plans. However, the family seemed determined to go ahead with the marriage, even though a deputy superintendent of police (DSP) visited the village and tried to prevent the marriage. The marriage did take place and no one was arrested. Worse still, villagers belonging to upper castes complained to the police accusing Bhanwari Devi of interference in their social customs. This resulted in social and economic boycott of Bhanwari and her family. The villagers stopped selling milk to the family or buying the earthen pots that she and her family made. Her husband was beaten up by Gurjar men in the village. But worst was yet to come.

At dusk on 22 September 1992, while Bhanwari and her husband were working in their field, five men from the dominant and affluent Gurjar caste from her village attacked her husband with sticks, leaving him unconscious. Thereafter, all five of them gang-raped her as a "punishment".

The accused were arrested and tried in the court, but they were backed by the local MLA.

How the Police and Medical Procedures Humiliated the Rape Victim?

Bhanwari Devi reported the incident to the *pracheta*, her block-level supervisor, who took her to the police station to lodge a first information report (FIR). The police showed extreme indifference and scepticism before lodging the FIR, a phenomenon very common in the Indian context. Scholars have recorded that all across South Asia "police are reluctant to record rape cases and show callousness and indifference towards women with complaints of rape". In this case Bhanwari Devi was asked to deposit her lehanga (long skirt) as evidence even though she had no other clothes to wear. She had to cover herself with her husband's blood-stained saafa (turban) and walk three kilometres to the nearest *saathin's* village, at an hour after midnight.

This indifference and humiliation continued at the Primary Health Centre (PHC) in the nearby town of Bassi, where no female doctor was present to medically examine Bhanwari Devi, and the male doctor refused to do so. He referred her to the district hospital in Jaipur, but wrote in his referral that she was being sent for a test "confirming the age of the victim." His report made no mention of the incident of rape.

The MO refused to conduct any tests without orders from a magistrate; the magistrate refused to give the orders until the next day, as it was past his working hours. As a result, the vaginal swab was taken more than 48 hours after the alleged rape, although Indian law requires this to be done within 24 hours. Scratches and bruises on her body were not recorded, and her complaints of physical discomfort were ignored.

How the Lower Judiciary too Harassed the Victim?

In a constitutional democracy, judiciary is the first and last hope for citizens seeking justice. Sadly, in this case, Bhanwari Devi's hope was shattered. Five judges hearing her plea were changed, and the sixth judge ruled that the accused were not guilty. He even observed that Bhanwari Devi's husband could not have passively watched his wife being gang-raped. The accused included an uncle-nephew pair, and the judge even said that a middle-aged man from an Indian village could not possibly have participated in a gang rape in the presence of his own nephew. He further stated that upper caste men cannot touch a lower caste woman, so the rape could not have taken place.

In 1995, the district and sessions court in Jaipur dismissed the case and acquitted all the five accused. An MLA organised a victory rally in the state capital, Jaipur, for the five accused who were now declared not guilty, and even members of the women's wing of his political party attended the rally calling Bhanwari Devi a liar.

However, a small report about her case appeared in newspapers, and this galvanised women's organisations all over Rajastan to come together. Women's activists and lawyers highlighted the fact that Bhanwari Devi attracted the ire of her rapists solely because of her work to create public awareness against child marriages. They filed a Public Interest Litigation (PIL) in the Supreme Court of India, under the collective platform of Vishakha, a **women's NGO**. The petition, filed by Vishakha and four other women's organizations in Rajasthan against the State of Rajasthan and the Union of India, resulted in what are popularly known as the Vishakha guidelines. The Supreme Court's judgment of August 1997 provided the basic definitions of sexual harassment at workplace and laid down the guidelines to deal with it.

Why was it necessary to give such a detailed background of Bhanwari Devi's plight and her fight for justice? It is because her story tells us how countless number of women in India suffer similar humiliation without getting justice from an insensitive social structure and an indifferent criminal-justice system. Ordinarily, a rape victim's constant humiliation by people belonging to powerful sections of society, police, hospital staff and the judiciary can make the person feel helpless and give up her efforts of getting justice. But in Bhanwari Devi's case, she was brave and determined even though she was utterly poor. She did not give up even when she had to sell everything she had in her pursuit of justice. Fortunately for her, she received support and solidarity from a group of women's organisations and socially committed lawyers, who took up the matter to the Supreme Court, which did not disappoint them. In the process, she won a great victory for millions of working women in India who suffer, mostly in silence, sexual harassment at workplace.

Sexual harassment at workplace is a menace that prevails everyday and everywhere all across India. It affects not only poor women belonging to "lower castes", but also rich and educated women belonging to "upper castes". It is not limited to any particular religion either. Sadly, our society was silent about this crime until the apex court issued legally binding guidelines to prevent it and also to bring the culprits to justice.

Bhanwari Devi received honours both nationally and internationally. She was invited to participate in the United Nations' Fourth World Conference on Women in Beijing in 1995. In 1994, she was awarded the **Neerja Bhanot Memorial Award** that carried a cash prize of ₹ 1 lakh for her "extraordinary courage, conviction and commitment". In 2002, the Chief Minister of Rajasthan allotted a residential plot to Bhanwari Devi and also announced a grant for construction of the house and for education of her son.

What do the Vishakha Guidelines Say?

The Vishakha guidelines include the following:

- A definition of sexual harassment
- Shifting accountability of women's safety from individuals to institutions
- Prioritizing prevention
- Provision of an innovative redress mechanism
- It is the impact and not the intent is to be considered.

The Supreme Court defined sexual harassment as any unwelcome, sexually determined physical, verbal, or non-verbal conduct. Examples include:

- Sexually suggestive remarks about women, comments, singing songs or whistling or winking while woman is passing by
- Demands for sexual favours
- Sexually offensive visuals in the workplace
- Use of the electronic media for harassment through sms, mms, videos, email, etc.

The definition also covered situations where a woman could be disadvantaged in her workplace as a result of threats relating to employment decisions that could negatively affect her working life. According to a handbook of the Government of India, "unwelcome behaviour" is experienced when the victim feels bad or powerless; and when it causes anger/sadness or negative self-esteem. The Government of India's handbook adds that **"unwelcome behaviour is one which is illegal, demeaning, invading the woman's privacy, one-sided and power based"**.

The Vishakha guidelines thus became a legal shield for self-defence for women at workplace in the absence of a law to provide for the effective enforcement of their basic human rights, gender equality and guarantee against sexual harassment and abuse.

'Nirbhaya' Case and New Laws to Check Sexual Crimes

Women's struggle for legal protection against sexual crimes achieved a new milestone when the central government was forced to enact a set of new laws in the wake of a gruesome incident of gang rape and murder in Delhi that shocked the nation on 16th December 2012. In response to what came to be known as the 'Nirbhya' case, the government enacted the following laws.

a. Criminal Law (Amendment) Act, 2013 (Nirbhaya Act)
b. Police reforms in management of cases related to crime against women
c. Sexual Harassment of Women at Workplace (Prevention, Prohibition and Redressal) Act, 2013.

With increased access to education and employment, millions of women are entering the country's workforce today. Many working women face sexual harassment at the workplace. It is crucial therefore to create a safe and secure environment for working women. The Sexual Harassment of Women at Workplace (Prevention, Prohibition and Redressal) Act, 2013 defined sexual harassment in clearer terms. It laid down the procedures for complaint and inquiry, and the action to be taken.

This Act provides a civil remedy to women and is in addition to other laws for women that are currently in force. The Act recognizes the **Right of every woman to a safe and secure workplace environment**, irrespective of her age or employment/work status. Hence, the right of all women working or visiting any workplace whether in the capacity of regular, temporary, ad hoc or daily wages basis is protected under the Act. **The law is entirely based on, and broadens the scope of, the Vishakha guidelines**. Thus, the law carries the spirit of the **Vishakha guidelines in terms of prohibition, prevention and redress**. These were the three key obligations that were imposed on institutions. In fact, the law mandates that every employer constitute an Internal Complaints Committee (ICC) at each office or branch office with approximate 10 or more employees. At least one member of the ICC has to be an outsider with experience in dealing with such cases. It is mandatory for every organisation to have the ICC; failure to set it up makes the organisation liable to be fined ₹ 50,000/-.

Women working in the informal sector, farm workers, domestic workers, and women working in shops, etc. can get redress from **local complaints committees**. These are to be formed at the district level under the district officer or the district collector. A woman can go to LCC even when the respondent is the head of the department or the head of the institute.

In this article we will concentrate only on the working of the Internal Complaints Committee.

EXAMPLES OF BEHAVIOURS AND SCENARIOS THAT CONSTITUTE SEXUAL HARASSMENT

Below are examples of behaviour that may or may not constitute workplace sexual harassment in isolation. At the same time, it is important to remember that more often than not, such behaviour occurs in cluster. <u>Distinguishing between these different possibilities is not an easy task and requires essential training and skill building</u>.

Some examples of behaviour that constitute sexual harassment at the workplace:

1. Making sexually suggestive remarks or innuendos.
2. Serious or repeated offensive remarks, such as teasing related to a person's body or appearance.
3. Offensive comments or jokes.
4. Inappropriate questions, suggestions or remarks about a person's sex life.
5. Displaying sexist or other offensive pictures, posters, mms, sms, whatsApp, or e-mails.
6. Intimidation, threats, blackmail around sexual favours.
7. Threats, intimidation or retaliation against an employee who speaks up about unwelcome behaviour with sexual overtones.
8. Unwelcome social invitations, with sexual overtones commonly understood as flirting.
9. Unwelcome sexual advances which may or may not be accompanied by promises or threats, explicit or implicit. Physical contact such as touching or pinching.
10. Caressing, kissing or fondling someone against her will (could be considered assault).
11. Invasion of personal space (getting too close for no reason, brushing against or cornering someone).
12. Persistently asking someone out, despite being turned down.
13. Stalking an individual.

14. Abuse of authority or power to threaten a person's job or undermine her performance against sexual favours.
15. Falsely accusing and undermining a person behind closed doors for sexual favours.
16. Controlling a person's reputation by rumour-mongering about her private life.

Some examples of behaviour that may indicate underlying workplace sexual harassment and merit inquiry

1. Criticizing, insulting, blaming, reprimanding or condemning an employee in public.
2. Exclusion from group activities or assignments without a valid reason.
3. Statements damaging a person's reputation or career.
4. Removing areas of responsibility, unjustifiably.
5. Inappropriately giving too little or too much work.
6. Constantly overruling authority without just cause.
7. Unjustifiably monitoring everything that is done.
8. Blaming an individual constantly for errors without just cause.
9. Repeatedly singling out an employee by assigning her with demeaning and belittling jobs that are not part of her regular duties.
10. Insults or humiliations, repeated attempts to exclude or isolate a person.
11. Systematically interfering with normal work conditions, sabotaging places or instruments of work.
12. Humiliating a person in front of colleagues, engaging in smear campaigns.
13. Arbitrarily taking disciplinary action against an employee.
14. Controlling the person by withholding resources (time, budget, autonomy, and training) necessary to succeed.

The above examples show two types of workplace harassments

1. *Quid Pro Quo*: Asking for sexual favours to offer promotion or some kind of benefit at workplace.
2. *Hostile work environment*: This is characterised by a work environment in which a women is subjected to lewd jokes, verbal abuse, and circulation of lewd rumours. She can complain of sexual harassment when she has grounds to believe that her objection would disadvantage her in connection with her employment or work including recruiting or promotion.

Internal Complaints Committee (ICC)

The law mandates that every organisation with 10 or more employees must set up an **internal complaints committee** or **ICC** to look into matters of sexual harassment of women at the workplace for the purposes of prevention, prohibition and redressal. It is the responsibility of every employer to ensure safety of all women in their work environment and to empower women for better and dignified participation in the work of the organisation. As mentioned earlier, the law defines various aspects of sexual harassment and protects all women working at, or even visiting, a workplace, in any capacity. It defines as "victim" any woman "of any age whether employed or not", who alleges to have been "subjected to any Act of sexual harassment".

After the amendment of the law in 2016, the **internal complaints committees** (ICC) are called internal committees (IC) only. Depending on the size of the organisation, the number of ICC members could be at least three and some times more than 6–7, but in larger organisations with varied stakeholders there can be committees with 10–12 members including or excluding an NGO member. ICC as per law will help women because:

1. It ensures a place where women employees could seek redress.
2. It sends a clear message to all the people at a workplace that there can be no compromise in matters of sexual harassment. It educates, trains and sensitises all employees in this regard. It also makes them aware that such complaints would be enquired into by a specially designated committee with external expertise.
3. It prevents a series of litigation that otherwise would follow in the absence of a workplace mechanism like the ICC.

Composition of the committee is given in Table 6.1.

Table 6.1: Composition of internal complaints committees (ICC)		
Sr. No.	ICC member	Eligibility
1.	Chairperson	Women working at senior level as employee; if not available then nominated from other office/units/department/workplace of the same employer.
2.	2 members minimum	From amongst employees committed to the cause of women/ having legal knowledge/experience in social work.
3.	NGO member	From amongst NGO/associations committed to the cause of women or a person familiar with the issue of sexual harassment.

Responsibilities of the organisation
- To form an internal committee and get all the members trained.
- To display, for awareness creation and training, IEC material created by the government or NGOs.
- The administration or management of the organisation cannot interfere with the working of the committee.

Importance of the NGO member in ICC: Section 4 Subsection (2) of the Sexual Harassment of Women (Prevention, Prohibition and Redressal Act, 2013 mandates for the appointment of an external member to the internal complaints committee. It says the external member should be a person from an NGO committed to the cause of women or a person familiar with issues related to sexual harassment.

Do's and don'ts for complaints committee	
Do's	Don'ts
1. Create an enabling meeting environment	1. Do not get aggressive
2. Use body language that communicates complete attention to the parties	2. Do not insist on a graphic description of the sexual harassment
4. Discard pre-determined ideas	4. Do not discuss the complaint in the presence of the complainant or the respondent
5. Determine the harm	5. Do not break the confidentiality at any cost

The role of the external member is crucial to the committee
- Provide hand holding support in the functioning of the ICC
- Assist the ICC in conducting the inquiry if/when there is a complaint.
- Record the minutes of the regular meetings.
- Prepare the content on the functioning of the ICC in the annual report of the organisation.
- Assist the employer in conducting awareness training for all the employees.
- Conduct orientation programme for the members of the ICC.
- Give appropriate advice as and when called for to the members of the ICC and to any employee who has approached.
- Ensure total compliance with the Sexual Harassment of Women at Workplace (Prevention, Prohibition and Redressal) Act, 2013.

External member should be
- Totally involved with all the ICC proceedings
- Must make sure that the proceedings are happening according to the principles of natural justice.
- Make efforts to coordinate the functioning of other ICC members.
- Ensure the implementation of law as per the procedures established.
- Ensure healthy and comfortable workplace and ensure that workplace harmony is restored in case of sexual harassment incidents.

Legal steps in resolving the complaint
Stage one: Receipt of the complaint.
Step 1: Receive and acknowledge receipt of the written complaint from the concerned woman, if she cannot write ICC to help her in the presence of NGO member.
Step 2: Meet and talk to the complainant (within eight days of getting complaint) to explore options for formal and informal resolutions.
Step 3: Informal mechanism if she says, that means she just wants the harassment to stop (if complainant agrees, take it in writing).
Step 4: Formal mechanism. Call the respondent with a confidential letter tell him about this complaint and give a copy of the complaint, ask for a written explanation (may give time for explanation and his list of witnesses).
Step 5: In case of formal complaint ask for any witnesses from the complainants also.

Stage two: List the witnesses, plan hearings, daytime
Step 1: Call witnesses with confidential letter.
Step 2: Recording who said what is important, inform the concerned persons, so that it is written verbatim.
Step 3: Write the minutes and send every one to check their portion.

Stage three: If any one of them complainant or respondents want to do the cross they are allowed to do so.
Step 1: Committee to come to conclusion depending on the circumstantial evidences, witnesses and respondent's response to the complaint, depending of probability of preponderance.
Step 2: Write the report in detail, with comments for every stage and step. List all the material submitted or created by the committee.
Step 3: Give recommendations as per the service rules, to the administrations.

Complete the enquiry in 90 days.

As per the law there is no internal appeal. Either complainant or the respondent who ever decides to go for appeal will have to go to the court or the tribunal.

Let us all have safe workplaces for women, let us all check if there are internal committees established by the administration.

Eliminating violence against women and advancing women's equality includes the right to be free from workplace sexual harassment.

REFERENCES

1. Policy against sexual harassment at workplace Municipal Corporation, Greater Mumbai 2004.
2. The Ministry of Women and Child Development Handbook on Sexual Harassment of Women at Workplace Act.
3. Google Images

Laws Pertaining to Sexual Abuse

Kruti Doshi

The Indian Penal Code contains mainly two laws, the POCSO Act and the Criminal Amendment Act, that pertain to sexual abuse that have been come into existence or gone through multiple amendments in last few years following the horrific Nirbhaya tragedy in 2012 and other incidents of child sexual abuse.

We are going to look at the provisions of the following Acts and their Amendments

1. The Protection of Children from Sexual Offences Rules (POCSO), 2012
2. The Criminal Law Amendment Act (Nirbhaya Act), 2013
3. The Criminal Law Amendment, 2018
4. The Protection of Children from Sexual Offences (POCSO) Bill, 2019.

The Protection of Children from Sexual Offences Rules, 2012
&
The Protection of Children from Sexual Offences Bill, 2019

Introduction

The Parliament has laid out a comprehensive legislation that gives importance to following aspects:

- **Protection of children** from the offences of sexual assault, sexual harassment and pornography
- **Safeguarding their interest** during judicial process
- **Child-friendly procedures** for reporting, recording of evidence, investigation and trial of offences
- Provision for establishment of **special courts** for speedy trial.

PROVISIONS OF POCSO ACT

- It extends to the whole of India, except the State of Jammu and Kashmir.
- Defines age and different forms of sexual abuse
- Stringent punishment graded as per the gravity of the offence
- Provides for mandatory reporting of sexual offences
- Casts the police in the role of child protectors during the investigative process
- Makes provisions for the medical examination of the child
- Provides for establishment of special courts.

Sexual Offences

Following are the offences described in the POCSO Act and the associated punishments. The Act was further amended by a Bill in 2019 and the changes in the Act are also described below.

A. Penetrative sexual assault

B. Aggravated penetrative sexual assault

C. Sexual assault

D. Aggravated sexual assault

E. Sexual harassment

F. Using a child for pornographic purposes

A. Penetrative Sexual Assault

A person is said to commit "penetrative sexual assault" if

- he penetrates his penis, to any extent, into the vagina, mouth, urethra or anus of child or makes the child to do so with him or any other person; or
- he inserts, to any extent, any object or a part of the body, not being the penis, into the vagina, the urethra or anus of the child or makes the child to do so with him or any other person; or
- he manipulates any part of the body of the child so as to cause penetration into the vagina, urethra, anus or any part of body of the child or makes the child to do so with him or any other person; or
- he applies his mouth to the penis, vagina, anus, urethra of the child or makes the child to do so to such person or any other person.

Punishment

Penetrative sexual assault (age of child)	POCSO Act punishment	Bill Amendment 2019 punishment
<16 years		20 years to life imprisonment with fine
>16 years	7 years to life imprisonment with fine	10 years to life imprisonment with fine

B. Aggravated Penetrative Sexual Assault

These include cases when a police officer, a member of the armed forces, a public servant, relative of the child commits penetrative sexual assault on a child or if the assault injures the sexual organs of the child or the child becomes pregnant.

The Bill adds two more grounds:

   i. Assault resulting in death of child

  ii. Assault committed during a natural calamity, or in situations of violence.

Punishment

Offence	POCSO Act punishment	Bill Amendment 2019 punishment
Aggravated penetrative sexual assault	10 years to life imprisonment and a fine	20 years imprisonment to death penalty

C. Sexual Assault

Whoever, with sexual intent touches the vagina, penis, anus or breast of the child or makes the child touch the vagina, penis, anus or breast of such person or any other person, or does any other Act with sexual intent which involves physical contact without penetration is said to commit sexual assault.

Punishment

Offence	POCSO Act punishment
Sexual assault	Shall not be less than **three** years but which may extend to **five** years, and shall also be liable to fine

D. Aggravated Sexual Assault

Includes cases where the offender is a police officer, member of the armed forces or security forces/public servant/the staff of a jail, or remand home/place of custody or care and protection, the management or staff of a hospital, the management or staff of an educational institution, gang sexual assault, sexual assault on a child using deadly weapons, fire, heated substance or corrosive substance, physically incapacitates the child, if the assault injures the sexual organs of the child, inflicts the child with human immunodeficiency virus, commits sexual assault on the child repeatedly/child <12 years/being a relative/being in the ownership or management or staff/being in a position of trust or authority of a child/the child is pregnant/makes the child to strip or parade naked in public.

- The Bill adds two more offences to the definition of aggravated sexual assault
    i. Assault committed during a natural calamity
    ii. Administrating or help in administering any hormone or any chemical substance, to a child for the purpose of attaining early sexual maturity.

Punishment

Offence	POCSO Act punishment
Aggravated sexual assault	Shall not be less than **five** years but which may extend to **seven** years, and shall also be liable to fine

E. Sexual Harassment

A person is said to commit sexual harassment upon a child when such person with sexual intent

- utters any word/sound/gesture or exhibits any object or part of body to be seen by the child; or
- makes a child exhibit his body or any part of his body so as it is seen by such person or any other person; or
- shows any object to a child in any form or media for pornographic purposes; repeatedly follows/watches child either directly or through any means; or
- threatens to use, in any form of media of any part of the body of the child or the involvement of the child in a sexual Act; or
- entices a child for pornographic purposes.

Punishment

Offence	POCSO Act punishment
Sexual harassment	Term of **three** years and shall also be liable to fine

F. Using a Child for Pornographic Purposes

A person is guilty of using a child for pornographic purposes if he uses a child in any form of media for the purpose of sexual gratification. The Act also penalises persons who use children for pornographic purposes resulting in sexual assault. The Bill defines child pornography as any visual depiction of sexually explicit conduct involving a child including photograph, video, digital or computer generated image indistinguishable from an actual child.

Punishment

Offence	POCSO Act, 2012	2019 Bill
Use of child for pornographic purposes	• Maximum: 5 years	• Minimum: 5 years
Use of child for pornographic purposes resulting in penetrative sexual assault	• Minimum: 10 years • Maximum: Life imprisonment	• Minimum: 10 years (in case of child below 16 years: 20 years) • Maximum: Life imprisonment
Use of child for pornographic purposes resulting in aggravated penetrative sexual assault	• Life imprisonment	• Minimum: 20 years • Maximum: Life imprisonment, or death
Use of child for pornographic purposes resulting in sexual assault	• Minimum: 6 years • Maximum: 8 years	• Minimum: 3 years • Maximum: 5 years
Use of child for pornographic purposes resulting in aggravated sexual assault	• Minimum: 8 years • Maximum: 10 years	• Minimum: 5 years • Maximum: 7 years

G. Storage of Pornographic Material

The Bill adds two other offences for storage of pornographic material involving children
  i. failing to destroy, or delete, or report pornographic material involving a child
 ii. transmitting, displaying, distributing such material except for the purpose of reporting it.

Punishment

Offence	POCSO Act punishment	Bill Amendment 2019 punishment
Storage of pornographic material	Up to 3 years of imprisonment and a fine	3 years to 5 years of imprisonment and a fine

Abetment of and Attempt to Commit an Offence

A person abets an offence, who
1. instigates any person to do that offence; or

2. engages with one or more other person or persons in any conspiracy for the doing of that offence, or

3. intentionally aids, by any Act or illegal omission, the doing of that offence.

Punishment

Whoever abets any offence under this Act, shall be punished with punishment provided for that offence.

Role of Medical and Health Professionals

1. Relevant Legal Provisions in the Act and Rules and related laws
2. Emergency medical care
3. Modalities of medical examination of children

1. Relevant Legal Provisions in the Act and Rules and Related Laws

A. *Section 27: Medical examination*
   a. To be conducted in accordance with Section 164A of the Code of Criminal Procedure, 1973
   b. The victim is a girl child, the medical examination shall be conducted by a woman doctor
   c. To be conducted in the presence of the parent of the child or any other person in whom the child reposes trust or confidence.

B. *Rule 5: Emergency medical care*
   a. Need of urgent medical care and protection
   b. No medical practitioner, hospital or other medical facility centre rendering emergency medical care to a child shall demand any legal or magisterial requisition or other documentation as a pre-requisite to rendering such care.
   c. Registered medical practitioner rendering emergency medical care:
      i. Treatment for cuts, bruises, and other injuries including genital injuries
      ii. Treatment for exposure to sexually transmitted diseases (STDs)
      iii. Treatment for exposure to human immunodeficiency virus (HIV)
      iv. Possible pregnancy and emergency contraceptives should be discussed with the pubertal child
      v. If necessary, a referral or consultation for mental or psychological health or other counselling
   d. Any forensic evidence collected in the course of rendering emergency medical care must be collected in accordance with Section 27 of the Act.

2. Emergency Medical Care

Section 23 of the Criminal Law Amendment Act, which inserts Section 357C into the Code of Criminal Procedure, 1973 provides that all hospitals are required to provide first-aid or medical treatment free of cost to the victims of a sexual offence.

A. *Medical examination*
   1. By a registered medical practitioner without delay and prepare a report of her examination giving the following particulars:
      • The name and address of the woman and of the person by whom she was brought;

- The age of the woman;
- The description of material taken from the person of the woman for DNA profiling; marks of injury, if any, on the person of the woman;
- [1]General mental condition of the woman.

2. The report shall state precisely the reasons for each conclusion arrived.
3. The report shall record that the consent of the woman or of the person competent to give such consent on her behalf to such examination had been obtained.
4. The exact time of commencement and completion of the examination be noted in the report.
5. The registered medical practitioner without delay forward the report to the investigation officer who shall forward it to the magistrate.
6. Nothing in this section shall be construed as rendering lawful any examination without the consent of the woman or of any person competent to give such consent on her behalf.

B. *Compensation for medical expenses*: Section 33(8) provides, in appropriate cases, the special court may, direct payment of such compensation as may be prescribed to the child for any physical or mental trauma caused to him or for immediate rehabilitation of such child.

Rule 7 specifies that the special court may order that the compensation be paid not only at the end of the trial, but also on an interim basis, to meet the immediate needs of the child for relief or rehabilitation at any stage after registration of the FIR.

3. Modalities of Medical Examination of Children

A. *Role of medical professionals in the context of the POCSO Act, 2012*
   a. Having an in-depth understanding of sexual victimization
   b. Obtaining a medical history of the child's experience in a facilitating, non-judgmental and empathetic manner
   c. Meticulously documenting historical details
   d. Conducting a detailed examination to diagnose acute and chronic residual trauma and STDs, and to collect forensic evidence
   e. Obtaining photographic/video documentation of all diagnostic findings that appear to be residual to abuse
   f. Formulating a complete and thorough medical report with diagnosis and recommendations for treatment
   g. Testifying in court when required

B. *Mandatory reporting*: When a doctor has reason to suspect that a child has been or is being sexually abused, he/she is required to report this to the appropriate authorities (i.e. the police or the relevant person within his/her organization who will then have to report it to the police).

Failure to do this would result in imprisonment of up to six months, with or without fine.

C. *Medical history*: Where a child is brought to a doctor for a medical examination to confirm sexual abuse, the doctor must:
   1. Take the written consent of the child. The three main elements of consent are information, comprehension and voluntariness.

2. Where the child is too young or otherwise incapable of giving consent, consent should be obtained from the child's parent, guardian or other person in whom the child has trust and confidence.
3. The right to informed consent implies the right to informed refusal.
4. To be able to give informed consent, the child and his/her parents/guardian need to understand that health care professionals may have a legal obligation to report the case and to disclose information received during the course of the consultation to the authorities even in the absence of consent.
5. Document who was present during the conversation with the child.
6. Document questions asked and child's answers in the child's own words.
7. Conduct the examination in a sensitive manner.
8. Focus on asking simply worded, open-ended, non-leading questions.
9. Using the child's words for body parts may make the child more comfortable with difficult conversations about sexual activities.
10. Using drawings may also help children describe where they may have been touched and with what they were touched.
11. The child has adequate privacy while the examination is being conducted.
12. Do not conduct the examination in a labour room.
13. Stop the examination if the child indicates discomfort or withdraws permission to continue.
14. Always prepare the child by explaining the examination and showing equipment;
15. If the child is old enough, and it is deemed appropriate, ask whom they would like in the room for support during the examination.
16. The medical history should cover any known health problems (including allergies), immunization status and medication.
17. Collect and preserve forensic evidence.
18. Clothing, especially underwear, is the most likely positive site for evidentiary DNA.
19. Scene investigation, including collection of linens and clothing should be done early.
20. Children often report weeks or months after the abuse event; consider differential diagnosis and alternative explanations for physical signs and symptoms.
21. In the case of a child with special needs, do not assume that the child will need special aid. Also, ask for permission before proceeding to help the child.

D. *Essentials in medical history*
   1. Last occurrence of alleged abuse
   2. First time the alleged abuse occurred
   3. Threats that were made
   4. Nature of the assault
   5. Whether or not the child noticed any injuries or complained of pain
   6. Vaginal or anal pain, bleeding and/or discharge following the event
   7. Any difficulty or pain with voiding or defecating
   8. Any urinary or faecal incontinence

E. *Essentials in medical examination*
   1. Record the height and weight of the child.
   2. Note any bruises, burns, scars or rashes on the skin. Carefully describe the size, location, pattern and colour of any such injuries.

3. Check for any signs that force and/or restraints were used, particularly around the neck and in the extremities.
4. Record the child's sexual development stage and check the breasts for signs of injury.
5. If the survivor is menstruating at the time of examination then a second examination is required on a later date in order to record the injuries clearly.
6. Record of whether the survivor was menstruating at the time of assault/ examination or bathing, douching, defecating, urinating and use of spermicide after the assault is important as some amount of evidence is lost.

F. *Role of medical professionals as expert witnesses*: Physicians can provide opinion testimony that is based upon the child's history, statements, and medical examination, even if the physician's examination of the child reveals no concrete physical evidence supportive of the child's allegations.

It is important to remember that the medical professional cannot be asked to testify to "diagnose" sexual abuse.

The doctor cannot make any definitive conclusions regarding the degree of force used by the abuser or whether the victim consented to any sexual activity.

What he/she can appropriately conclude is whether there is evidence of sexual contact and/or recent trauma. He/she can state whether the medical history and examination are consistent with sexual abuse.

It is important to remember that while an expert's testimony may be deemed relevant, necessary, reliable, and therefore admissible under the aforementioned guidelines, it is ultimately the prerogative of the judge to determine what weight should be afforded the testimony.

THE CRIMINAL LAW (AMENDMENT) ACT, 2013—NIRBHAYA ACT

The Criminal Law (Amendment) Bill, 2013 commonly known as the Anti-rape Bill came into force on April 3, 2013. Thereafter, this Bill called The Nirbhaya Act, 2013.

Historical Context

- Need for a strict law to deal with sex crimes against women was felt after the brutal gang-rape and murder of a 23-year-old paramedical student in a moving bus in the national capital on December 16, 2012.
- Brutality of the crime shocked the nation and Indians protested on the streets to demand better safety measures for women and strict laws to punish the culprits.
- Under public pressure, Congress-led UPA government at the Centre formed Justice JS Verma panel to come up with strict laws to arrest crime against women.

Key Points in The Nirbhaya Act, 2013

- Law maintains life imprisonment for rape as the maximum sentence, yet sets down the death penalty for repeat offenders and those whose victims are left in a "vegetative state".
- Expands the meaning of rape to include penetration of the mouth, anus, urethra or vagina with the penis or any other object without consent.
- Defines stalking and voyeurism as crimes with punishments up to seven years.

- Gang rape has been recognized as an offence, while sexual harassment has been redefined to include unwelcome advances with sexual overtures and showing pornography without consent.
- The age of consent of sex has been kept at 18.
- Law also punishes police and hospital authorities with imprisonment of up to two years if they fail to register a complaint or treat a victim.

Provisions of the Criminal Law (Amendment) Act, 2013—Nirbhaya Act

The following sections were added to the Criminal Law Amendment Act.

Section	Offence	Punishment	Notes
326A	Acid attack	Imprisonment not less than ten years but which may extend to imprisonment for life and with fine which shall be just and reasonable to meet the medical expenses and it shall be paid to the victim	Gender neutral
326B	Attempt to acid attack	Imprisonment not less than five years but which may extend to seven years, and shall also be liable to fine	Gender neutral
354A	Sexual harassment	Rigorous imprisonment up to three years, or with fine, or with both in case of offence described in clauses (i), (ii) or (iii) Imprisonment up to one year, or with fine, or with both in other cases	Only protects women. Provisions are: i. Physical contact and advances involving unwelcome and explicit sexual overtures; or ii. A demand or request for sexual favours; or iii. Making sexually coloured remarks; or iv. Forcibly showing pornography
354B	Act with intent to disrobe a woman	Imprisonment not less than three years but which may extend to seven years and with fine	Only protects women against anyone who "Assaults or uses criminal force to any woman or abets such Act with the intention of disrobing or compelling her to be naked"
354C	Voyeurism	In case of first conviction, imprisonment not less than one year, but which may extend to three years, and shall also be liable to fine, and be punished on a second or subsequent conviction, with imprisonment of either description for a term which shall not be less than three years, but which may extend to seven years, and shall also be liable to fine	Only protects women. By implication, women may prey voyeuristically upon men with impunity
354D	Stalking	Imprisonment up to three years for the first offence, and shall also be liable to fine and for any subsequent conviction would be liable for imprisonment up to five years and with fine	Only protects women from being stalked by men. By implication, women may stalk men with impunity

Criticisms of the Law

Law has been severely criticized for:

- Being gender biased and giving women the legal authority to commit exactly the same crimes against men with impunity.
- Not including certain suggestions recommended by the Verma Committee Report like, marital rape, reduction of age of consent, amending Armed Forces (Special Powers) Act so that no sanction is needed for prosecuting an armed force personnel accused of a crime against woman.

THE CRIMINAL LAW (AMENDMENT) ACT, 2018

An Act to further amend the Indian Penal Code, Indian Evidence Act, 1872, the Code of Criminal Procedure, 1973 and the Protection of Children from Sexual Offences Act, 2012 was brought about in 2018.

Section	Offence	Punishment	Cognizable	Bailable	Court trial
376	Rape	Imprisonment of not less than 10 years may extend to imprisonment for life and with fine	Cognizable	Not bailable	Court of session
376	Rape by a police officer or a public servant or member of armed forces or by staff of a jail/remand home/women's or children's institution or by staff of a hospital rape or by a person in a position of trust or authority or by a near relative	Imprisonment of not less than 10 years may extend to imprisonment for life and with fine	Cognizable	Not bailable	Court of session
376	Persons committing offence of rape on a woman under sixteen years of age	Imprisonment of not less than 20 years may extend to imprisonment for life and with fine	Cognizable	Not bailable	Court of session
376AB	Persons committing offence of rape on a woman under 12 years of age	Imprisonment of not less than 20 years may extend to imprisonment for life and with fine or with death	Cognizable	Not bailable	Court of session
376DA	Gang rape on a woman under 16 years of age	Imprisonment for life and with fine	Cognizable	Not bailable	Court of session
376DB	Gang rape on a woman under 12 years of age	Imprisonment for life and with fine or with death	Cognizable	Not bailable	Court of session

SOURCE REFERENCES AND SUGGESTED READING

1. The Ministry of Law & Justice; The POCSO Act, 2012 (No. 32 of 2012).
2. The Ministry of Law & Justice; The Criminal Law Amendment Act, (Nirbhaya Act) 2013.
3. The Ministry of Law & Justice; The Criminal Law Amendment Act, 2018 (No. 22 of 2018).
4. The Ministry of Law & Justice; The Protection of Children from Sexual Offences Bill, 2019.
5. Ministry of Women & Child Development Model Guidelines under Section 39 of The Protection of Children from Sexual Offences Act, 2012.
6. www.child_sexual_abuse_laws_in_India.

POCSO and Practitioners

Jaydeep Tank

Background: Bareilly rape survivor denied abortion: Progressed to 32 weeks.

- **July 26:** Girl's family moves petition before lower court for abortion
- **August 4:** They approach fast trackcourt with the petition.
- **August 13:** Court declines permission.
- **August 22:** Teenager's family moves application before HC for termination of pregnancy.
- **August 29:** Court asks girl's father to move application before chief medical officer (CMO).
- **September 3:** Victim's counsel meets CMO, who allegedly declines to Act.
- **September 5:** Family approaches district magistrate.
- **September 12:** Doctors that reviewed the pregnancy turn down request for medical termination.

Talking Points

- Do adolescents have sex and need contraception?
- Which contraception method is suitable?
- The law and adolescent sexuality.

Sheer weight of numbers[1]

- The World Health Organisation (WHO) estimates that about 33% of the Indian population, or about 300 million, is in the age group of 10–24 years, and adolescents (10–19 years) form about 70% of the 10–24 age group—210 million adolescents. The difference between the genders is primarily on account of the difference in the ages at which they tend to get married. Most sexual encounters in India tend to be of the conjugal kind, the data suggests. Thus, women tend to have sex at an earlier age because they get married at a younger age (Figure 8.1).

  Nearly half—**45%**—of young women in India marry (begin cohabiting with their husband) **before** age **18**, the legal age at marriage for women. A majority, **63%**, marry **before** age **20**. Yet, there has been a **slow trend toward delaying marriage:** Nationally, the proportion of women marrying before their 18th birthday declined by five percentage points from 1993 to 2006, from 50% to 45%.

- Contraceptive use remains very **low**: Just 7% of married 15–19-year-old women use a modern method, and 6%, a traditional method. Current use of modern methods ranges from a high of 18% in Delhi to a low of 2% in Bihar.

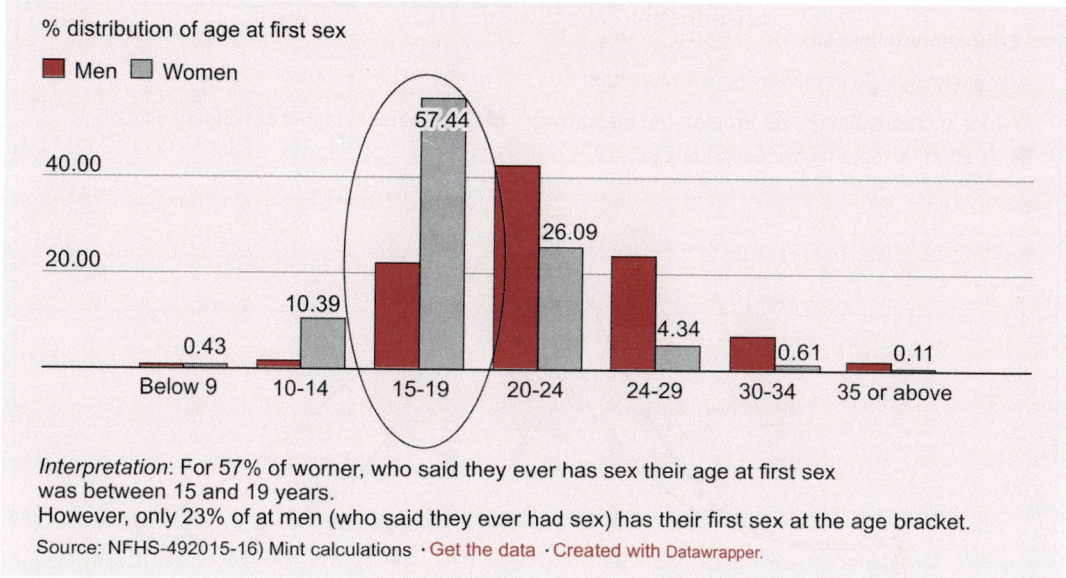

% distribution of age at first sex

■ Men ☐ Women

Interpretation: For 57% of worner, who said they ever has sex their age at first sex was between 15 and 19 years.
However, only 23% of at men (who said they ever had sex) has their first sex at the age bracket.
Source: NFHS-492015-16) Mint calculations · Get the data · Created with Datawrapper.

Figure 8.1: Age at first coitus

- **Forty-three percent** of married 15–19-year-old women have an unmet need for modern contraception, down considerably from 52% in 1993, but still a very high proportion.
- Unplanned childbearing among adolescents is not uncommon: **14%** of all adolescents' recent births were **unplanned** in 2006, a proportion that remained basically unchanged from that in 1993.
- Pre-marital sexual activity among adolescents is considerable, is not coerced in a majority and is not influenced by residential or educational status (Figure 8.2).[2]
- Most adolescents begin their sexual activity **without adequate knowledge** about sexuality or contraception or **protection** against STIs/HIV.
- For **unmarried** adolescents it is sometimes impossible to access contraceptives and the sexual activity often results in unintended pregnancy.
- Whether married or unmarried, adolescents face potentially serious physical, psychological and social consequences from **unprotected** sexual relations, ranging from early and unwanted pregnancy and childbirth, unsafe abortion to STIs including HIV/AIDS.

Barriers to contraceptive use among adolescents[3]
- The unexpected and unplanned nature of sexual activity
- Lack of information and knowledge about conception and contraceptives and their availability.
- Fear of medical procedures
- Fear of judgemental attitudes of providers
- Inability to pay for services and transport
- Fear of opposition from partner or parents
- Pressure to have children.
- Care providers are unaware and insensitive to the special needs of adolescents.

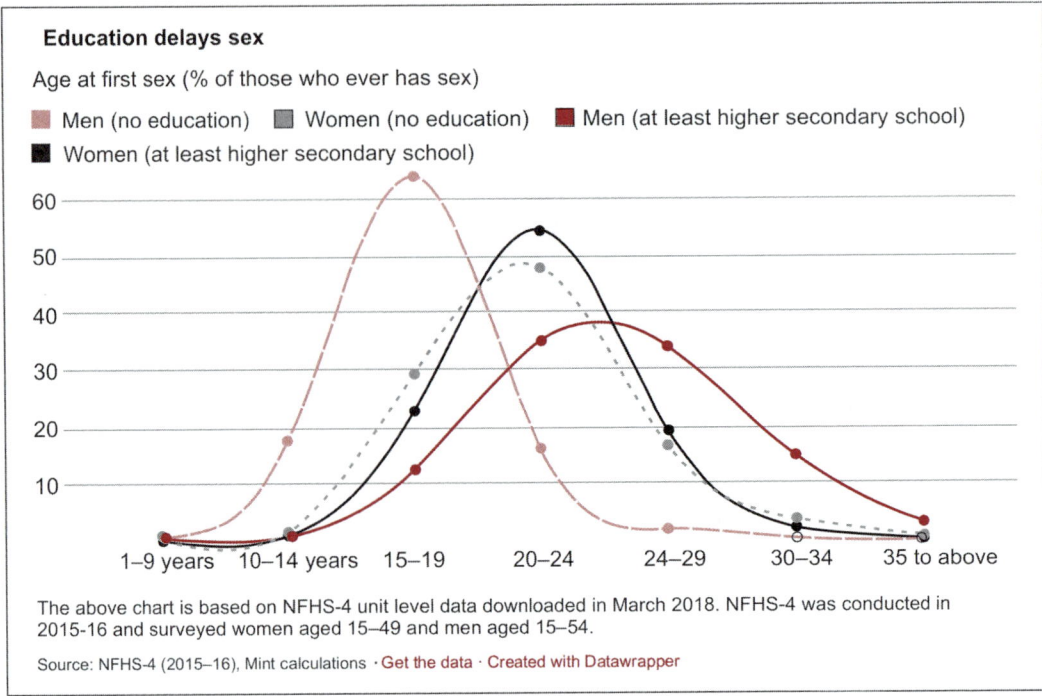

Education delays sex

Age at first sex (% of those who ever has sex)

- Men (no education) ■ Women (no education) ■ Men (at least higher secondary school)
- Women (at least higher secondary school)

The above chart is based on NFHS-4 unit level data downloaded in March 2018. NFHS-4 was conducted in 2015-16 and surveyed women aged 15–49 and men aged 15–54.

Source: NFHS-4 (2015–16), Mint calculations · Get the data · Created with Datawrapper

Figure 8.2: Effect of education on sex

- They need to overcome their attitudes and moral and tradition-related biases and respond to the special needs of adolescents by designing and reorienting health services to meet those needs.
- Health care providers need to also be aware of gender inequalities that alienate and marginalize adolescent girls in their communities and prevent them from seeking technically skilled care.
- Perceptions are shaped by teaching, experience and media.

Does the knowledge and availability of contraception increase promiscuity? No COCs[4]

- 10–15% of adolescents on hormonal contraception still get pregnant.
- Discontinuation rates for hormonal contraception in young girls are high, with many girls complaining about side effects, particularly breakthrough bleeding.

Emergency Contraception

- Progestin-only OCPs containing the hormone levonorgestrel can be used for emergency contraception. If the correct dose is started within 72 hours after unprotected intercourse, it reduces the chances of pregnancy.
- Now oral contraceptives are being packaged as emergency contraceptive pills, and levonorgestrel-only tablets are more effective and cause less nausea and vomiting.
- Emergency contraception has a special role for adolescent girls and women who are subjected to sexual violence, to prevent unwanted pregnancies.
- There is a need to increase access to ECPs by training healthcare providers and also by ensuring easy availability of ECPs. All adolescents are eligible for ECP, without restriction on repetitive use.

The Protection of Children from Sexual Offences (POCSO) Act, 2012

- Section 2(1)(d) defines a "child"—as any person below the age of 18 years.
- The criminalisation of all sexual activity below the age of 18 years
- Any person (including a child) can be prosecuted for engaging in a sexual Act with a child irrespective of whether the latter consented to it.
- The Act does not recognize consensual sexual Acts among children or between a child and an adult.
- Under Section 19 of the POCSO Act, 'Reporting of offences' by any person including the child has been made mandatory.
- Section 21 of the Act provides punishment for failure to report or record a child sexual abuse case. However, a child cannot be punished for failure to report {S.21 (2)}.

Abetment (Section 16)

- A person abets an offence, who
  - *First*: Instigates any person to do that offence; or
  - *Secondly*: Engages with one or more other person or persons in any conspiracy for the doing of that offence, if an Act or illegal omission takes place in pursuance of that conspiracy, and in order to the doing of that offence; or
  - *Thirdly*: Intentionally aids, by any Act or illegal omission, the doing of that offence.
- The Act is gender neutral.
- Before the Act was passed, debates took place around the need to acknowledge and decriminalise sexual behaviour of adolescents between 12 and 18 years.
  - The Act, however, adopted an approach under the assumption that a uniform age of consent would be in accordance with the UN Convention on the Rights of the Child, 1989.
- In effect, the Act infringes upon the right to dignity and bodily integrity, freedom of expression, right to life, and the right to privacy of adolescents engaging in consensual sexual behaviour.[6]

The National Commission for Protection of Child Right (NCPCR) had stressed on the need for the law to recognise consensual sexual exploration among adolescents by decriminalising it when it is between:

- Children above 12 years when the age gap was less than two years
- Children above 14 years when the age gap was less than three years.

By not recognising this, the POCSO Act has conflated adolescent sexuality with child sexual abuse.

It has failed to consider nuances of age, age difference, and child development.

Conflict and Conflation

Section 3

- Notwithstanding anything contained in the Indian Penal Code (45 of 1860), a registered medical practitioner shall not be guilty of any offence under that Code or under any other law for the time being in force, if any pregnancy is terminated by him in accordance with the provisions of this Act.
- Subject to the provisions of sub-Section (4), a pregnancy may be terminated by a registered medical practitioner.

- Where the length of the pregnancy does not exceed twelve weeks if such medical practitioner is, or where the length of the pregnancy exceeds twelve weeks but does not exceed twenty weeks, if not less than two registered medical practitioners are, of opinion, formed in good faith, that
    i. The continuance of the pregnancy would involve a risk to the life of the pregnant woman or of grave injury to her physical or mental health; or
    ii. There is a substantial risk that if the child were born, it would suffer from such physical or mental abnormalities to be seriously handicapped.

Explanation 1: Where any pregnancy is alleged by the pregnant woman to have been caused by **rape**, the anguish caused by such pregnancy shall be presumed to constitute a grave injury to the mental health of the pregnant woman.

Explanation 2: Where any pregnancy occurs as a result of **failure of any device or method** used by any married woman or her husband for the purpose of limiting the number of children, the anguish caused by such unwanted pregnancy may be resumed to constitute a grave injury to the mental health of the pregnant woman.

Explanation 3: In determining whether the continuance of a pregnancy would involve such risk of injury to the health as is mentioned in sub-Section (2) account may be taken of the pregnant womens **actual or reasonable foreseeable environment**.

Explanation 4: (a) No pregnancy of a woman, who has not attained the age of **eighteen years**, or, who, having attained the age of eighteen years, is a **mentally ill person**, shall be terminated except with the consent in writing of her guardian? (b) Save as otherwise provided in clause (a), no pregnancy shall be terminated **except with the consent** of the pregnant woman.

Section 5

- Sections 3 and 4 when not to apply
- (1) The provisions of Section 4, and so much of the provisions of sub-Section (2) of Section 3 as relate to the length of the pregnancy and the opinion of not less than two registered medical practitioners, shall not apply to the termination of a pregnancy by a registered medical practitioner in a case where he is of opinion, formed in good faith, that termination of such pregnancy is immediately necessary to save the life of the pregnant woman.
- Section 5 of the Act gives obstetricians or even nonobstetricians the ability to terminate the pregnancy in the interest of the mother's life irrespective of the period of gestation.
- The Government needs to emphasise this that in most cases health—defined as mental or physical health—can provide sufficient justification for the termination of pregnancy. The Government thus need not modify the law but simply give guidance or interpretation of this section.
- In case of foetal abnormalities the agony and issues of mental health of the woman who is forced to carry a foetus with lethal or severe abnormalities (grave mental harm), along with the fact that termination at any time of pregnancy is safer than delivery at term (particularly for adolescents and young girls) can also justify termination under Section 5.
- Recommendation would be to "seek for a better and more inclusive interpretation of Section 5 of the MTP Act".

Does a provider have a legal duty to inform the authorities if a minor girl is pregnant? Yes

- A pregnant minor girl married/unmarried is considered a victim of sexual assault, and a medical provider is required to report the pregnancy to the appropriate authorities, even if the girl has not expressed a desire to take legal action.
- Marital status makes no difference to the reporting requirement under the POCSO Act.
- If the girl's age is uncertain, it is advised to report the pregnancy as per the legal requirement under the POCSO Act and to allow the authorities to decide what actions to take.
- The provider does not need to wait for the authorities to take action and may proceed with the termination of pregnancy in line with the provisions of the MTP Act after maintaining complete and detailed records of the case.

What conduct is sufficient to satisfy a provider's duty to report under the POCSO Act while offering MTP services to a minor?

- The National Commission for the Protection of Child Rights (NCPCR) has stated that providing a medico-legal certificate to the authorities is sufficient to comply with the reporting requirements of the POCSO Act.[7]

Does a medical provider have to wait for any medico-legal procedure before performing the abortion? No

- Rule 5(3) of the POCSO Rules states that "no medical practitioner, hospital or other medical facility centre rendering emergency medical care to a child shall demand any legal or magisterial requisition or other documentation as a pre-requisite to rendering such care."
- Similarly, the 2013 Ministry of Health and Family Welfare Guidelines and Protocols: Medico-legal Care for Survivors/Victims of Sexual Violence state, "Providing treatment and necessary medical investigations is the prime responsibility of the examining doctor" and that "admission, evidence collection or filing a police complaint is not mandatory for providing treatment."
- Rape is a legal ground for terminating a pregnancy under Section 3 of the MTP Act up to 20-week of gestation. After 20 weeks, abortion is permissible under Section 5 of the MTP Act, if the provider is of the opinion that it is necessary to terminate the pregnancy to save the life of the woman.
  - **Therefore, it is important to provide medical care at the earliest while legal proceeding can continue simultaneously.**
  - It is unnecessary to approach the authorities for permission to terminate an adult or minor rape survivor's pregnancy within the permissible first 20 weeks as defined under the MTP Act, or thereafter, if such termination is required to save her life.

Does the medical provider have a legal obligation to preserve the products of conception for abortion services for minor girls? Not always

- Section 201 of the Indian Penal Code prohibits causing "any evidence of the commission" of an offence to disappear with the intention of screening the offender from legal punishment.
- Crucially, Section 201 includes an important intent component. It would be considered a violation under Section 201 only if a provider destroys evidence with the intent to protect the accused from legal action.

- Therefore, providers who dispose of the products of conception (PoC) for a good faith reason (inadequate preservation facilities, or following standard operating procedures, for example), should be shielded from prosecution under Section 201.

Protection for Providers

- Section 8 of the MTP Act guarantees protection for providers who Act in good faith.
- This clause recognises that above all else, it is imperative that girls and women receive the highest standard of medical care available.
- Accordingly, all providers should fulfill their reporting requirements and legal obligations under the MTP Act and the POCSO Act after ensuring essential services.

> **PMO**
> *"The question of adolescent sexuality should not be an issue in the political arena. When a woman (girl) has to make these kinds of decisions, she should see her doctor, not her lawyer."*

What we must do?[8,9]

- Move from a one-size-fits-all approach to one that responds to the varying needs of different groups of adolescents.
- Expand the range of contraceptive choices offered to adolescents from 'condoms only' to the full range of methods.
  - Move away from separate health services for adolescents, and instead make existing health services that already serve adolescents, to some extent, more adolescent-friendly, e.g. antenatal clinics, postnatal clinics, STI/HIV clinics, and as extensions to under-five clinics.
- Work more actively with pharmacies and shops to expand contraceptive access and uptake, as our current focus on public health facilities alone does not fully reflect where adolescents obtain their contraceptives.
- Move from one-off in-service training for a handful of providers to a package of actions to ensure that all levels of health workers, including support staff, respond to adolescent clients effectively and with sensitivity.
- We must provide adolescents with comprehensive sexuality education (CSE) in an age and developmentally-appropriate manner.

SOURCE REFERENCES AND SUGGESTED READING

1. Ann M. Moore, Susheela Singh, et al. Adolescent Marriage and Childbearing in India: Current Situation and Recent Trends. Guttmacher Foundation, April 2009.
2. Sonia Trikha. Indian Journal of Community Medicine, Vol. 26, No. 1, 2003.
3. RKSK (RashtriyaKishorSwasthyaKaryakram), MOHFW, GOI.
4. Clark, L. (2004). Journal of Adolescent Health, 34 (2), 123–124.
5. AAP recommendations. http://www.contemporarypediatrics.com/modern-medicine-featurearticles/contraception-guidelines-adolescents.
6. Gupta, N., Corrado, S., and Goldstein, M. (2008). Pediatrics in Review, 29 (11), 386–397.
7. http://www.tarshi.net/inplainspeak/voices-love-andsex-in-the-time-of-the-pocso-Act-2012/
8. http://ncpcr.gov.in/showfile.php?lang=1&level=1&&sublinkid=406&lid=843
9. Chandra-Mouli, et al. Reproductive Health (2017) 14:85.

MTP in Survivors of Sexual Assault: Medico-legal Challenges

Nikhil D Datar

Introduction

Medical Termination of Pregnancy (MTP) Act was passed in 1971. The provisions of the Indian Penal Code, more particularly Section 312 stated that the termination of pregnancy was a criminal offence. The MTP Act carved out an exception to the Indian Penal Code. Thus, MTP Act, although selectively, allows women to undergo termination of pregnancy legally. Pregnancy arising out of sexual assault is one of the legitimate grounds for termination of pregnancy. Section 3(2) B) (i) of MTP Act states that if the continuance of the pregnancy involves a risk to the life of the pregnant woman or grave injury to her physical or mental health, it is a valid indication for MTP.

In fact, the honourable Supreme Court of India in cases of Miss X and Dr Nikhil Datar *vs* Union of India allowed the termination of pregnancy at 24 weeks. This was the first successful case in the country wherein termination was allowed beyond 20 weeks of pregnancy. After this case, the author helped more than 150 women to file cases for termination of pregnancy (ToP). These cases paved way for the proposed amendment to the existing Act.

In day-to-day practice, a gynaecologist is challenged by many practical situations. Various laws such as the MTP Act, Indian Penal Code, Criminal Law Amendment Act, Protection of Children from Sexual Offences (POSCO) Act pose classic medico-legal challenges. Moreover, right to privacy and right for medical treatment can put the doctor in catch 22 situation.

In this article the author has taken an account of such situations.

Can MTP under Section 3(2) (B) (i) be done only after the rape is proven?

The explanation 1 under the MTP Act reads as under:

Where any pregnancy is alleged by the pregnant woman to have been caused by rape, the anguish caused by such pregnancy shall be presumed to constitute a grave injury to the mental health of the pregnant woman.[1]

Thus, it is clear that even, if the woman has alleged rape, it is enough to proceed with MTP.

What is the maximum gestational age at which MTP can be done for rape survivor?

The author believes that MTP should be allowed at any gestation in cases of rape survivors as long as the procedure is not going to pose excessive risk to the survivor's life/health.

- At this point of time, the MTP Act (1971) allows TOP only up to 20 weeks.
- The MTP amendment bill of 2020 proposes to raise the limit to 24 weeks.

The author was instrumental in helping a 12-year-old rape survivor to file a case for MTP beyond 20 weeks. The Supreme Court allowed termination of pregnancy at 31 weeks of gestation. The same was successfully carried out at JJ Hospital, Mumbai. This seems to be the highest gestational age so far, at which court have allowed termination of pregnancy.[2]

What is the current state of the amendment of MTP Act?

At this point of time, the Ministry of Health and Family Welfare, Government of India has proposed the amendment bill in the ongoing session (March 2020) of parliament. It is expected that the bill will be passed without any resistance. After the bill will be passed, the Ministry of Health and Family Welfare will frame the rules and regulations. The government will notify date of implementation in the official gazette. On or after the said date the amended law will be applicable in the country.

What special precautions should be taken when the Registered Medical Practitioner (RMP) undertakes to do MTP for a rape survivor?

Given that the survivor is a woman above the age of 18 and is of sound mind to consent for the procedure, a woman may approach the doctor in one of the following manners:
1. The woman has already filed a case in the police station. In that case the police will bring her for evaluation and treatment including MTP.
2. The woman may directly approach the RMP with a request for MTP.
3. The woman may bring the order of the court.

Scenario 1: The doctor should ensure whether or not the basic examination and collection of evidence has been done. Usually in this case the examination and evidence collection would have been done already. After adequate medical investigations the procedure for MTP may be undertaken. The police should be kept in loop so that products of conception can be handed over for DNA analysis in sealed container. This is an important piece of evidence to prove the offence.

If examination and evidence collection has not been done beforehand, the doctor should elaborately record the details. The Ministry of Health and Family Welfare, Government of India in 2014 has released the document titled "Guidelines and Protocols: Medico-legal care for survivors/victims of sexual violence".[3]

Since the assault will not be a recent one, there is no point in collecting multiple swabs as prescribed in the proforma. Scientific facts such as spermatozoa cannot be identified after 72 hours of the assault must be borne in mind while conducting such examination.

The author has come across a case where the woman was pregnant because of an assault nearly 2 months back but she was recently assaulted again. In such a case elaborate collection of samples will have to be done. The RMP is guided by the history given by the woman.

Consent taking in case of examination of survivor

The consent is to be taken for:

a. Medical examination for treatment
b. Medico-legal examination
c. Sample collection for clinical and forensic examination.

A woman has a right of refusal to consent to any of the above. Her refusal must be recorded in writing.

Scenario 2: The woman may approach the doctor directly for MTP and give history of sexual assault. She may request the doctor to provide the medical treatment/MTP but may not want to file a police complaint.

This raises a vital ethical-legal question: **What should be the response of the RMP when survivor of sexual assault requests for TOP but is not willing to file police complaint?**

As a general rule, any serious crime (cognizable offence) must be reported to the police. Section 39 (1) of Code of Criminal Procedure 1973, casts duty to inform the police officer or magistrate when the person is aware of commission or intent of "certain" offences. Interestingly this list of "certain offences" does not mention the offences related to sexual assaults. Thus, it may be construed that the RMP is not duty bound to inform about sexual assault especially when the woman does not want to initiate any legal proceedings. However, this theory has not yet been tested in any legal proceedings so far.

The practice of informing the police when there is a knowledge of alleged sexual assault prevails. The police machinery also expects that the same is adhered to. The guidelines from the Government of India[3] have laid down the following mechanism while dealing with such a situation.

- It is expected that the doctor makes a medico-legal case in any event.
- The woman must be informed about her right to refuse filing an FIR.
- She cannot be forced to undergo examination/evidence collection by police or court.

Scenario 3: If the woman comes to the doctor with the order of the court, the doctor has to follow the order in its entirety.

Should the MTP be done only in government hospital?

The Criminal Law Amendment Act 2013, in Section 357C Criminal Procedure Code states that both private and public health professionals are obligated to provide treatment. Denial of treatment of rape survivors is punishable under Section 166B IPC with imprisonment for a term which may extend to one year or with fine or with both.

This abundantly clarifies that the TOP can be done in private sector as well.

What safeguard is there for the RMP who provides MTP to an adult unmarried woman who later on claims that the said pregnancy was out of sexual assault?

Such incidences have been reported although very rarely. In most of these incidences it has been found that the man had falsely promised marriage and had engaged into sexual intercourse leading to pregnancy. Later on the man refused to keep up the promise.

Whatever the social factors may be, the RMP should take elaborate history before providing the services. The RMP, if in doubt, may confirm the age of the woman by asking for age proof. The RMP may take abundant precaution by requesting the woman to write a letter stating that the said pregnancy is not out of sexual assault. This absolves him from potential harassment in the hands of police.

What are the medical standards of care for providing MTP?

Ministry of Health and Family Welfare, Government of India has provided medical guidance in its document "Comprehensive Abortion Care: Training and Service Delivery Guidelines". The second edition of the same was released in 2018. The RMPs may refer to these as standard guidelines while providing MTP services to rape survivors.[4]

What are the legal provisions when providing MTP to minors?

Protection of Children from Sexual Offences (POCSO) Act was passed in 2012 in India with a specific purpose. The Act defines "child" as any person below the age of eighteen years. A child does not have capacity to consent. Thus, sexual intercourse with a child automatically becomes an assault and thus a criminal office. Thus, when a minor girl comes to the RMP for MTP, it is mandatory for the RMP to inform the police. In fact, failure to do so may attract imprisonment for six months and/or fine. Since the minor does not have capacity to consent, the parents' consent has to be obtained for termination of pregnancy.

Does the reporting to the police against the woman's wish violate the privacy of the individual?

Honourable Supreme Court of India in 2017 gave a landmark judgement stating that privacy is fundamental right of individuals.[5]

If an adult survivor of sexual assault wishes not to file a police complaint, the same should be respected. The RMP should record her refusal to inform the police in writing and proceed with the treatment. The customary practices are in contradiction to this. This poses a complex situation for the medical professional.

In case of women between the aged sixteen and eighteen another challenge comes up. Many of these girls express that the sexual encounter was "consensual" in nature. Usually the partner is nearly of the same age. Being a consensual intercourse they do not want to report to the police but only want the MTP. On the other hand, the RMP is duty bound to inform the police under POCSO. Once the police machinery comes into play and the teenaged male is arrested. The knowledge of this arrest becomes public and it strips the young female and male's privacy too which POCSO sought to enshrine.

Secondly, when a woman is made aware that the case will be informed to the police they do not come forward for the treatment. Thus, medical treatment is also indirectly denied by mandatory reporting of such cases.

In a recent case in 2019, the Madras High Court while acquitting a young accused of charges under POCSO made some important suggestions. It was suggested that the definition of "child" under Section 2D of POCSO Act should be redefined as 16 instead of 18. Secondly, consensual sex after the age of 16 should decriminalised or be tried under liberal provisions.

CONCLUSION

Medical termination of pregnancy in rape survivor poses complex ethical and legal situations. Complexity of law, namely POCSO, CLA pose challenging medico-legal scenario for the RMP. There is immediate need to provide medico-legal protection to the RMP so that the RMP can concentrate on medical treatment of survivors instead of getting hassled with legal provisions.

REFERENCES

1. [Online] [Cited: 5 march 2020.] https://mohfw.gov.in/Acts-rules-and-standards-health-sector/Acts/mtp-Act-1971.
2. [Online] [Cited: 5 march 2020.] https://www.bbc.com/news/world-asia-india-41172796.
3. Ministry of health and family welfare government of India. [Online] [Cited: 4 march 2020.] https://mohfw.gov.in/sites/default/files/953522324.pdf.
4. https://nhm.gov.in/New_Updates_2018/NHM_Components/RMNCHA/MH/Guidelines/CAC_Training_and_Service_Delivery_Guideline.pdf. [Online] [Cited: 5 march 2020.] https://nhm.gov.in/New_Updates_2018/NHM_Components/RMNCHA/MH/Guidelines/CAC_Training_and_Service_Delivery_Guideline.pdf.
5. [Online] [Cited: 5 march 2020.] https://www.npr.org/sections/thetwo-way/2017/08/24/545963181/indian-supreme-court-declares-privacy-a-fundamental-right.

Marital Rape

Jyothi Unni, Kruti Doshi

Marital rape is defined as an Act of sexual intercourse without the spouse's consent. It need not involve violence, but is considered a form of domestic violence and sexual abuse. It is mostly experienced by women, but men can also be victims of rape within marriage.

Marital rape has been impeached in more than 100 countries but, unfortunately, India is one of the only 36 countries where marital rape is still not criminalized.

Historically, when a couple was married, it was presumed that this meant consent for sexual intercourse. It was felt that lawful marriage legitimizes the conjugal Act, so a spouse cannot withdraw that right.

When activists started fighting for human rights and gender equality, they challenged this supposition. In 1993, the United Nations declared marital rape a human rights violation.[1] A statement declared "and that is rape, when a man forces himself sexually upon a woman, whether he is licensed by the marriage law to do it or not."

Status of Marital Rape in India

- The **definition of rape codified in Section 375** of the Indian Penal Code (IPC) includes all forms of sexual assault involving non-consensual intercourse with a woman.
- Non-criminalization of marital rape in India emanates from **Exception 2 to Section 375** which exempts unwilling sexual intercourse between a husband and a wife over fifteen years of age from Section 375's definition of "rape" and thus immunizes such Acts from prosecution. This exception has been modified to include sexual Acts between spouses, provided the wife is not under the age of 18. This has been done since the Protection of Children from Sexual Offences Act, 2012 (POCSO)[2] protects girls between the ages of 15 and 18.
- As per current law, a wife is presumed to deliver perpetual consent to have sex with her husband after entering into marital relations.
- The concept of marital rape in India is the epitome of what we call an "implied consent". Marriage between a man and a woman here implies that both have consented to sexual intercourse and it cannot be otherwise.
- Under Section 376B, marital rape is a crime, if sexual intercourse by the husband takes place during separation and if the woman is below 18 years of age.

Marital Rape: Against Legal and Constitutional Rights

1. **Doctrine of Coverture**
   - Non-criminalised nature of marital rape emanates from the British era. The marital rape largely influenced by and derived from this doctrine of merging the woman's identity with that of her husband.
   - At the time the IPC was drafted in the 1860s, a married woman was not considered an independent legal entity.
   - The marital exception to the IPC's definition of rape was drafted on the basis of Victorian patriarchal norms that did not recognize men and women as equals, did not allow married women to own property, and merged the identities of husband and wife under the **"Doctrine of Coverture"**.

2. **Violation of Article 14:** Marital rape violates the right to equality enshrined in Article 14 of the Indian Constitution.[3]
   - The exception creates two classes of women based on their marital status and immunizes actions perpetrated by men against their wives.
   - In doing so, the exception makes possible the victimization of married women for no reason other than their marital status while protecting unmarried women from those same Acts.

3. **Defeats the Spirit of Section 375 of IPC:** The purpose of Section 375 of IPC is to protect women and punish those who engage in the inhumane activity of rape.
   - However, exempting husbands from punishment is entirely contradictory to that objective, as the consequences of rape are the same whether a woman is married or unmarried.
   - Moreover, married women may actually find it more difficult to escape abusive conditions at home because they are legally and financially tied to their husbands.

4. **Violation of Article 21:** According to interpretation by the Supreme Court, rights enshrined in Article 21[4] include the rights to health, privacy, dignity, safe living conditions and safe environment, among others
   - In the State of Karnataka *vs* Krishnappa, the Supreme Court held that sexual violence apart from being a dehumanizing Act is an unlawful intrusion of the right to privacy and sanctity of a female. In the same judgment, it held that non-consensual sexual intercourse amounts to physical and sexual violence.
   - In the Suchita Srivastava *vs* Chandigarh Administration, the Supreme Court equated the right to make choices related to sexual activity with rights to personal liberty, privacy, dignity, and bodily integrity under Article 21 of the Constitution.
   - In Justice KS Puttuswamy (Retd.) *vs* Union of India, the Supreme Court recognized the right to privacy as a fundamental right of all citizens.
   - The right to privacy includes "decisional privacy reflected by an ability to make intimate decisions primarily consisting of one's sexual or procreative nature and decisions in respect of intimate relations.
   - In all these judgements the Supreme Court has recognized the right to abstain from sexual activity for all women, irrespective of their marital status, as a fundamental right conferred by Article 21 of the Constitution.

Therefore, forced sexual cohabitation is a violation of the fundamental right under Article 21.

Marital rape has come under public scrutiny in recent times. And what's worse, data on marital rape exists. It is being recorded by the National Family Health Survey (NFHS), which is a government run survey. NFHS 4, conducted in 2015–2016 reports that it occurs in 5.4% of marriages. It also notes that 31% of married women are subjected to physical, sexual or emotional violence and that the husband was the perpetrator in 83% of those who were sexually abused.[5]

Legal Remedies for Marital Rape

- Women can file complaints about sexual assault under Section 498A against their husbands.
- Protection of Women from Domestic Violence Act, 2005.[6] Under the Act, women can file complaints against forced sexual activity without their will, even by their spouses.

The increasing rate of crimes against women indicates the shortcomings of the present laws. The duty of safeguarding women's rights is not confined to the judiciary; it must be imbibed in the collective conscience of the nation.

Way Forward

The **United Nations Declaration on the Elimination of Violence against Women** (DEVAW) defines violence against women as "any Act of gender-based violence that results in, or is likely to result in, physical, sexual, or mental harm or suffering to women, including threats of such Acts, coercion or arbitrary deprivation of liberty, whether occurring in public or private life."[7]

In 2013, the UN Committee on Elimination of Discrimination against Women (CEDAW) recommended that the Indian government should criminalize marital rape.

The **JS Verma Committee** set up in the aftermath of nationwide protests over the December 16, 2012 gang rape case had also recommended the same.[8]

It is high time that the legislature should take cognisance of this legal infirmity and bring marital rape within the purview of rape laws by eliminating Section 375 (Exception) of IPC which will make women safe from abusive spouses, also help them to recover from marital rape and save themselves from domestic violence and sexual abuse.

Rape is rape, irrespective of the identity of the perpetrator, and age of the survivor. A woman, who is raped by a stranger, lives with a memory of a horrible attack; a woman who is raped by her husband lives with her rapist. Our penal laws handed by the British have by and large remained untouched even after 73 years of independence despite English laws being amended and making marital rape a criminalizing Act way back in 1991.

We can only hope that government will soon pass a law criminalizing marital rape.

REFERENCES

1. UN Commission on Human Rights, World Conference on Human Rights., 9 March 1994, E/CN.4/RES/1994/95, available at: https://www.refworld.org/docid/3b00f08c30.html.
2. The Ministry of Law & Justice; The POCSO Act, 2012.

3. The Article 14 of Constitution of India, 1949.

4. The Article 16 of Constitution of India, 1949.

5. National Family Health Survey 4 (NFHS-4)-2015-2016-International Institute for Population Sciences, Deonar, Mumbai 400008, Ministry of Health and Family Welfare.

6. Protection of Women from Domestic Violence Act, 2005 published by Ministry of Law and Justice.

7. Declaration on the Elimination of Violence against Women—UN Documents: Gathering a body of global agreements". Un-documents.net. Retrieved February 24, 2010.

8. Report of the committee on amendments to criminal law. [Accessed on February 12, 2019]. Available from: http://www.prsindia.org/uploads/media/Justice%20verma%20committee/js%20verma%20committe%20report.pdf.

Medico-legal Tips in Case of Sexual Offences

Amit Karkhanis, Jyoti Kukreja

Abstract

The Act of touching a person without his/her consent is a crime and punishable under the criminal laws of India. However, in order to obtain evidence against the accused for any sexual offence alleged to be committed by him, legal procedures fall back on medicine. The documented findings by the Registered Medical Practitioner (RMP) form a pivotal evidence of the case. The forensic medicine helps the victim and the court to expedite the trial and bring justice to the society. Since the reforms in the criminal laws allow the victim of sexual offence to approach the RMP without filing an FIR makes the RMP more vulnerable and prone to medico-legal cases. Hence, for RMPs to provide their services legally, it is important for them to be aware about the Laws, Rules and Regulations of treating and examining the victims of sexual offence. This article aims to discuss the steps, caution and measures that must be taken by an RMP before examining the victim.

Introduction

The World Health Organisation (WHO) defines sexual violence as "any sexual Act, attempt to obtain a sexual Act, unwanted sexual comments/advances and Acts to traffic, or otherwise directed against a person's sexuality, using coercion, threats of harm, or physical force, by any person regardless of relationship to the victim in any setting, including but not limited to home and work." A sexual offence has been defined by the Law Reform Commission of Canada (1978) as sexual contact with another person (including touching of the sexual organs of another) or touching of another with one's sexual organs without that person's consent. Any person may understand sexual violence as any sexual Act using coercion regardless of their relationship to the victim, in any setting, including but not limited to home and work. In sexual violence, coercion constitutes an important component, which covers a whole spectrum of degrees of force. Apart from physical force, it may involve psychological intimidation, blackmail or other threats (Bancroft, J., 1974).[1]

India recorded an average of 87 rape cases daily in 2019 and overall 4,05,861 cases of crime against women during the year, a rise of over 7% from 2018.[2] Whenever a man penetrates or does sexual intercourse with a woman without her consent, it amounts to rape. Section 354 of IPC criminalises any Act by a person that assaults or uses criminal force against a woman with an intention or knowledge that it will outrage her modesty. Section 354A of IPC defines sexual harassment. Rape can result into various extragenital injuries, psychological symptoms, STDs, pregnancy, etc. Such incidents can leave psychological impacts on the mind of the victim such as sleep problems, anger, guilt, etc. Section 53(5) of the CrPC states about examination of a female victim, which should be done by or under the supervision of a female doctor. Section 53A of the CrPC provides for a detailed medical examination of a person accused of an offence of rape or an attempt to commit rape. It sets down the requirements of medical examination of a person accused of rape.

Physical Examination of the Victim

Immediate physical examination of the victim is most important since the examination is the beginning point of any investigation. Furthermore, it helps in ruling out the possibility of false allegation, which happens many times because of many reasons. In India, though about 80% of the rape cases are charge sheeted by the police, a large number of these cases ultimately end in acquittal because of various factors like delayed reporting, unfavourable medical opinion, witnesses turning hostile, etc. One important factor behind the failure of a huge number of cases of rape in courts of law is the negative or false opinion provided by the Medical Practitioners who examine the rape victims. Medical evidence is one of the vital evidences to establish the fact that the victim was raped. The police investigator relies on the Medical Practitioner who examined the victim for collecting the finest evidence in the case— evidence from the body parts of the victim. The Law Commission in its Report (1980) had pointed out that "the report of medical examination is often cursory or is not sent in time". The Commission recommended some additions to the provisions in the Code of Criminal Procedure, the most important being that the "report shall state precisely the reasons for each conclusion arrived at".[3] The report shall include whether the sexual Act was completed or attempted, how recent was the offence on the victim committed, age of the victim and whether the victim was intoxicated with alcohol or drugs.

Sexual offences have a long-term impact on the physical as well as mental well-being of the victim. In such cases, the victim possesses the fundamental right to be treated without discrimination. Right to health, though not explicitly mentioned in the constitution of India, has been interpreted to be a part of right to life enshrined under Article 21 of the Constitution of India. Right to health is also enshrined in various international instruments ratified by India, including the International Covenant on Economic, Social and Cultural Rights (ICESCR), the Convention on the Elimination of Discrimination against Women (CEDAW), the Convention of the Rights of the Child (CRC), and the Convention on the Rights of Persons with Disabilities (CRPD).

Role of Examining Medical Practitioner in Providing Health Care to the Victims

Section 164(A) of the Criminal Procedure Code expressly states the legal obligations of the examining RMP in cases of rape. Section 27(1) of POCSO Act states that the medical examination of a child in respect of whom any offence has been committed under this Act, shall also be conducted in accordance with Section 164A of the Code of Criminal Procedure, 1973.

- Examination of the victim shall be conducted by a registered medical practitioner (RMP) employed in a hospital run by the government or a local authority and in the absence of such a practitioner, by any other RMP.
- Examination must be conducted without delay and an analytic report should be prepared by the RMP. Consent should be obtained explicitly for this examination. The consent form must be signed by the person himself/herself if she/he is above 12 years of age. Consent must be taken from the guardian/parent if the survivor is under the age of 12 years or if the survivor is unable to give his/her consent by reason of mental disability (Section 89 of IPC).
- Exact time of start and close of examination should be recorded.

  Even if the survivor refuses consent to submit evidence to the Forensic Science Laboratory (FSL) and reveal information to the police for purposes of investigation, she should be made aware that if at a later date she changes her mind and wants to pursue a legal course of action, the collected evidence may be useful to seek justice.
- RMP must forward the medical report of the victim without any delay to investigating officer (IO), and in turn IO to magistrate.[3]

  The RMP must attempt to create a good rapport with the victim. The RMP must refrain himself/herself from forming judgements or expressing disbelief with regards to victim's case or the incident explained by the victim. The duty of the RMP is to provide treatment to the victim just as any other patient. The RMP cannot discriminate the victim based on her caste, religion, profession, reliability on the victim's story, etc. Even sex worker reserves the right to decide with whom he/she will have sex with and non-consensual sexual intercourse even with a sex worker amounts to rape. The RMP must not assume that since the victim is a sex worker, he/she must be a sex addict or HIV positive. The RMP must document the information with respect to sexual intercourse complained of and not the past encounters as evidences.

In the case of *State of Karnataka vs Manjanna*,[4] it was held that medical examination of rape victims is a **"medico-legal emergency"**. It is the right of every victim and a duty of every hospital to medically examine the victim before filing of a legal complaint, and the hospital at the request of the victim, can afterwards file a complaint. A hospital may receive a victim of rape when victim voluntarily reports to the hospital, on requisition by the police or by the court.

However, POCSO Act provides for mandatory reporting of sexual offences against children, so that any adult, including a doctor or other health care professional, who has knowledge that a child has been sexually abused is obligated to report the offence. To supplement the procedure laid in Section 164A, after the Nirbhaya case, Ministry of Health and Family Welfare in 2014 gave certain guidelines and protocols for medico-legal care for the victims of sexual violence:

1. Basic details and consent: The medical examiner shall record the name, age, address, sex, name and relationship of the person who brought the rape victim/survivor and the consent of the victim.
2. Before taking the consent of the victim, victim shall be informed of the nature of medical examination. Only in life-threatening cases, the doctor may proceed with the examination without the consent as given in Section 92, IPC.
3. Identification marks: Two marks of identification should also be recorded, e.g. moles, scars or any mark.

4. Menstrual and vaccination history is to be recorded, and if the victim is menstruating at the time of the examination then a second examination is required on a later date in order to record the injuries clearly.

5. History of incidence: Medical examiner shall record the history of the incidence in survivor's own words, which shall have evidentiary value in court of law. If the history is narrated by a person other than the survivor, his/her name shall be noted.

6. Details of the clothing, medical and surgical history should be recorded.

7. General physical examination: Response to doctor's questions, space and time awareness, pulse rate, blood pressure, temperature, pupil and stain or semen mark on the clothes of the victim should be examined and recorded.

8. Examination of injuries: The entire body surface should be examined for any injuries, fractures, nail abrasions, teeth bite marks, cuts, boils, lesions, any discharge, weapon infection or stain on the body and shall be recorded with particular details of these injuries.

9. Examination of genital parts and orifices: External genital area and perineum is observed for evidence of injury, seminal stains, stray pubic hair, and foreign material. Sample of pubic hair and matted pubic hair is taken and preserved.

10. Examination of vagina is done with the help of sterile speculum lubricated with warm saline/ sterile water to check the internal bleeding, bruises or any injuries. Such examination is not required in cases of minor where there are no signs of penetration or visible injuries. If at all the examination is required, it shall be done under the effect of anaesthesia.

11. Two-finger test: Per vaginum examination must not be conducted for establishing rape/sexual violence and the size of the vaginal introitus has no bearing in a case of sexual violence. The guideline was given after the Supreme Court's judgement which held that the test is a violation of a woman's right to privacy. The two-finger test is a way to determine whether the hymen of the woman is intact or not. It is based on the assumption that hymen can rupture only when a female undergoes sexual intercourse. The method is unscientific, against human rights and has no bearing on determination of commission of rape.

12. Any injury, swelling, bleeding, discharge or stain near anus, anal opening and oral cavity should be examined and recorded.

13. Collecting samples: If requested by police, radiographs of wrist, elbow, shoulders, dental examination, etc. are be advised to be collected for age estimation.

14. Urine sample: To determine the pregnancy.

15. Blood test: Blood sample is collected for evidence of baseline HIV status, VDRL and HbsAg.

16. Post examination: After examination, medical practitioner should document the report, formulate opinion and sign the report. A copy of report must be given to the survivor, as it is her right to know about the information.

17. All the evidences collected during the examination, like clothes of the woman, swabs from vagina, anal opening, etc. pubic hair sample, foreign material, nail scrapings, swab sticks along with the report must be placed in an envelope and handed over to the police or judicial magistrate.

In landmark judgment of *Delhi Commission of Women v. Delhi Police*,[5] mandated certain changes in the police system, health services, child welfare committees, legal services and support services in order to give justice to victims of rape. The court pronounced that a SAFE Kit (Sexual Assault Forensic Evidence collection Kit) be used by all medical personnel for gathering and preserving physical evidence following sexual assault.

Sexual Assault Under POCSO Act

It is important for the doctor to remember that child sexual abuse is often a diagnosis based on medical history, rather than on physical findings. The medical history will guide the physical examination. Its objective is not to obtain information for forensic purposes but for treatment and diagnosis and to ensure the safety of the child.

Interviewing Techniques Under POCSO Act

The interview should begin by assessing the child's competence. This can be done by asking questions unrelated to the abuse, such as favourite colours, school activities, and likes and dislikes.

- The interview should not have an investigative tone. Relevant questions need to be asked to obtain a detailed paediatric history.
- Determine child's verbal and cognitive abilities, level of comfort, and attention.
- Document the questions asked and the child's responses verbatim, take a note of the body language, demeanour and emotional responses to questioning.
- Detailed medical history, past incidents of abuse or suspicious injuries, and menstrual history should be documented.
- Ask the child to identify body parts; including names for genitalia and anus (use an anatomically appreciate diagram). Write the findings on the diagram in detail.
- Ask about different types of touch; include kisses, hugs, tickles, spankings, and pinches or bites. Use the diagram to ask about all possible abusive touches and ask about any other times (places) it happened.
- It is best to avoid leading and suggestive questions; instead, maintain a "tell-me-more" or "and-then-what-happened" approach. Avoid showing strong emotions such as shock or disbelief.[5]

CONCLUSION

In every case involving sexual abuse or child abuse, an RMP has to provide his professional service with utmost caution and without discrimination. Above all, health workers should aim to convey the truth of what they saw and concluded, be it in a written report or to the court, in an impartial way, and ensure that a balanced interpretation of the findings is given.

REFERENCES

1. Sex Related Offences and their Prevention and Control Measures: An Indian Perspective by Dr. Barindra N. Chattoraj
2. https://thewire.in/women/average-87-rape-cases-daily-over-7-rise-in-crimes-against-women-in-2019-ncrb-data
3. Guidelines & Protocols Medico-legal care for survivors/victims of Sexual Violence http://biharpolice.bih.nic.in/ORDER-2019/MoH&FW%20guidelines%20on%20medicolegal%20care%20for%20rape%20victims.pdf
4. 2000 (3) SCR 1007
5. Manual for Manual for Manual for Medical Examination of Medical Examination of Medical Examination of Sexual Assault. http://pldindia.org/wp-content/uploads/2013/04/Manual-for-medical-examination-of-Sexual-Assault-CEHAT.pdf

Multidisciplinary Responsibilities

Responsibilities of Health Care Providers to Address Gender-based Violence

Nayreen Daruwala

Gender-based violence (GBV), including violence against women and children by both intimate and non-intimate partners, is both a violation of human rights and a global public health issue.[1] Worldwide, 15–71% of women suffer physical, psychological or sexual intimate partner violence at some point.[2] Globally one in three women have faced violence intimate partner violence and sexual violence by non-intimate partner. In South Asia, 42% of women have suffered violence by intimate partner at some point in their lives. In India, 29% of women have reported domestic violence in the last year.

Violence causes non-fatal or fatal injuries: 21% of homicides in southeast Asia are committed by an intimate partner, constituting 60% of all female homicides (the figure for male homicides is 1%).[3] Other harms to health include sexually transmitted infections, miscarriage, induced abortion, stillbirth, low birth weight, preterm delivery, harmful drug and alcohol use, anxiety and depression, self-harm, suicide, and trans-generational recapitulation of violence.[4-6] Physical and psychological trauma and fear lead to mental health problems, limited sexual and reproductive control, somatoform conditions, 4 difficulties in seeking health care, and lost economic productivity.[7] Violence is associated with male authority over female behavior, justification of wife beating, and women's economic disadvantage,[8] all of which are manifest in India. Intimate partner violence is endemic, domestic violence extends beyond the WHO definition,[9] to culturally sanctioned household maltreatment,[10] and non-partner sexual violence is reported regularly in the media.[11]

A systematic review of prevalence and health effects of violence against women carried out by WHO confirms that women undergo varied health effects due to violence.[12] 17 papers were identified, reporting on 16 studies, giving a total of 36, 163 participants, and containing 55 effect estimates showed a positive direction of effect between violence and depression and suicide. The review identified a total of 37 studies, providing 77 estimates of association between physical and/or sexual intimate partner violence and alcohol use.

41 studies carried out in the systematic review included cohort control, case control and cross-sectional studies from Africa and India showed an association between experience of intimate partner violence and biologically confirmed incident HIV and other STIs. In this review on global prevalence of intimate partner homicide, a survey of 169 countries with official data sources showed the median prevalence of intimate

partner homicide was approximately 13%, with as many as 38% of all murdered women (in contrast to 6% of all murdered men) being killed by an intimate partner. The median prevalence of intimate partner homicide among all murdered women was highest in the South East Asia Region, with approximately 55%, and the high-income region, with approximately 41%, followed by the African Region (40%) and the Region of the Americas (38%).[13]

Hospitals are often first place for disclosing violence. All women are likely to come in contact with health services at some point in their lives. Women subjected to violence are more likely to seek health services in general, often for conditions linked to violence, even if in most cases they do not disclose the violence. Health services provide a unique resource to identify women subjected to violence, provide them with appropriate care, connect them to other support services and, potentially, contribute to preventing future harm.

Health systems have a critical role in the multisectoral response in:

1. Early identification of women experiencing violence, providing appropriate care and referrals, providing them (and their children) with comprehensive health services.
2. Facilitating access to supportive services in other sectors that women who experience violence need and want.

Health care provider's approach to women survivors of violence is instrumental in providing them care and support. The role of health care providers needs to move from building forensic evidence to initiating therapeutic processes. The role is not limited to clinical assessment and treatment, but in making the woman comfortable to share her experience and enable her to seek support.

This is achievable if the care and health services for women who have been subjected to violence are women-centered that is, they should be organised around women's health needs and perspectives.

A women-centered health response offers care that
- takes actions to enhance women's safety;
- minimizes or does no harm and maximizes benefits of how services are designed and delivered;
- takes into account women's perspectives;
- responds to women's needs and concerns in humane and holistic ways;
- provides women with information and supports them to make informed choices and decisions;
- **empowers women to participate in their own care**.

World Health Organisation has described a rights-based approach for women wherein she has the right to live a violence free life of self-determination and non-discrimination. She has the right to attain the highest standard of health. On the other hand, it explains the responsibilities of the health care providers to work with a rights-based approach. The health care providers need to prioritise the survivor's right to privacy and confidentiality, right to relevant information and right to be treated fairly without any discrimination. The World Health Organisation has laid down protocols for pathways to treatment. The first-line response by health care providers is to listen sensitively, inquire about her needs and concerns, validate her feelings briefly, enhance her safety and extend her support by referring her to counseling services. It is important for health care providers to take informed consent, ensure consultation in a private space and ensure confidentiality. Once initial support is provided, clinical interventions and documentation play an important role in supporting the survivor's pathway to care.

There should be absolute confidentiality, and information should only be shared with other professionals if there is a real risk to the woman's life, a child is being abused, or a person discloses that they intend to harm or kill someone else. While it is always preferable to do this with the consent of the woman, in some cases it may be necessary to do this without her consent. However, she should always be informed of what information is being shared, with whom and why.[14]

The protocols put a lot of emphasis on documentation stating that health care professionals must document cases accurately and meticulously without judgement. They should not interpret what the woman says, but provide an accurate account of what she says and what is observed by the health professional (e.g. injuries, etc.). The medical record should be kept somewhere confidential and should not be accessible to the perpetrator or family members.

It is also very important to consider the referrals provided to the woman. There are situations where the survivor is in crisis and has little knowledge about what can be done, or there are situations where the survivor is unwilling to seek support. The health care provider's role in making referrals is influential for the survivor to seek help. Referring the survivor to another agency without an explanation may not help her to access services. But in cases of warm referrals the survivor gets the confidence to seek services.

Cold referral: A 'cold referral' involves providing information about another agency or service so that the client can contact them.

Warm referral: A 'warm referral' involves contacting another service on the client's behalf and may also involve writing a report or case history of the client for the legal service and/or attending the service with the client.

- Speaking directly to the service you are referring the person to and checking it is appropriate for them.
- Introducing yourself and the person to the referring agency and providing a verbal and/or written handover (with the person's consent).
- Developing a referral pathways list for the service that identifies and shares useful contacts.
- Following up with the person to see how the referral is working out.
- Getting support from colleagues to help identify appropriate services for referrals in particular locations or for specific issues.

It is important to explore with women how their children are being treated by the perpetrator, in a nonjudgmental way.

Children living in domestic violence situations should not always be interpreted as child abuse and will not necessarily require mandatory reporting. Each case must be assessed individually in order to make a judgement. Mandatory reporting of all cases can result in unintended harmful consequences. This form of reporting may deter women from disclosing violence and could jeopardize their safety. However, it is also important to recognize that persistent witnessing of serious forms of domestic violence is a child-protection issue.[14]

"In order to be sustainable, efforts to improve the response of the health system to GBV need to target several levels: The level of the actual health care provider (staff level), the level of health facilities, such as hospitals, clinics, health centres or doctor's practices (management level), and the level of health policy (policy makers and public administration)".[15]

SNEHA has initiated **Women's Out Patient Departments (OPDs)** in three tertiary hospitals and one teaching hospital as a full-time service with crisis counseling and referral systems in co-ordination with different departments. Primary prevention is done through trainings conducted with all levels of health care providers to make them understand the issue of violence against women and children. Secondary and tertiary interventions are provided through counseling and extended response to the survivors of violence. This has helped us in standardising protocols across all hospitals to provide a comprehensive package of care. The response to violence in women's lives is strengthened with a holistic approach that addresses women's immediate and long-term needs, recognises the emotional trauma they may suffer and challenges the stigma that accompanies gender-based violence.

In addition to referring cases to hospitals, we also receive referrals from the hospital. If through the course of treatment physicians recognise that the patient needs counseling or is a survivor of violence, then they write a note and refer them to the women's OPD. The counselors keep the doctor in the loop about the case throughout subsequent interventions, which includes social investigation, counseling, legal support, rehabilitation, and providing shelter if necessary. Based on the survivor's consent, SNEHA counselor calls the perpetrator and the necessary family members for the counseling process. A total of 5,566 cases have been registered in all the OPDs since their inception. 75% of cases have been of intimate-partner and domestic violence, 15% of sexual violence and 10% of child sexual abuse cases registered under POCSO.

Creation of an enabling environment is very crucial for health care provider's "buy-in" to respond to gender-based violence. National policies and procedures need to be place, as it may be difficult to work in an environment where laws and policies do not recognize violence against women as a problem or may even sanction, e.g. men "disciplining" their wives. Trainings should focus on increasing the core motivation of clinicians to effectively respond to the health care needs of their patients and this can be linked to the prevalence and health consequences of VAW. Partnerships between the health care sector and other statutory bodies and NGOs are critical to the success of VAW interventions, since many women will present with complex multiple needs.

Broadening the scope to include all forms of VAW helped to engage health care professionals. This approach also facilitates linkages between the intervention programme and a range of national policies and legislative frameworks. A core-group of health care professionals intensively trained on regular basis promotes a sense of ownership of the work and their roles within the system.

Surveillance tends to focus on injury and will not provide accurate information about the health burden of violence. Other approaches are needed to get a more complete picture of the problem. There is a need for more research on the effectiveness of interventions in relation to outcomes for women and children, as well as on their cost effectiveness.

A systemic responsiveness is crucial which implies that policy, strategy and practice is located within a framework of rights and state accountability. Specifically, the initiatives within the health systems should not singularly be attached to individual functionaries to address specific needs of the survivors; instead initiatives at the systems level should be supported institutionally by mandates, clear policy guidelines and protocols. The health systems' responsiveness could be examined along a continuum of 'prevention and response' interventions in 'addressing IPV' including—recognition and voicing of the issue, identification of vulnerabilities, facilitating referrals and institutional linkages, and creating an enabling environment. The systematic responsiveness is a matter of public policy and governance and can be unpacked by working on an intentional design rather than an incidental design.

REFERENCES

1. UN Millennium Project. Taking action: achieving gender equality and empowering women. New York: Task force on education and gender equality, 2005.
2. Devries KM, Mak JY, Garcia-Moreno C, et al. The global prevalence of intimate partner violence against women. Science 2013; 340: 1527–8.
3. Kilonzo N, Dartnall E, Obbayi M. Briefing paper: policy and practice requirements for bringing to scale sexual violence services in low resource settings. Nairobi: LVCT and SVRI, 2013. 13
4. What Works. A summary of the evidence and research agenda for What Works: a global programme to prevent violence against women and girls. Pretoria: UK Aid, 2014.
5. Remme M, Michaels-Ibokwe C, Watts C. Approaches to assess value for money and scale up of violence against women and girls prevention: a summary of the evidence. Pretoria: UK aid, 2014.
6. Pronyk PM, Hargreaves JR, Kim JC, et al. Effect of a structural intervention for the prevention of intimate-partner violence and HIV in rural South Africa: a cluster randomised trial. Lancet 2006; 368(9551): 1973–83.
7. Jewkes R, Nduna M, Levin J, et al. Impact of stepping stones on incidence of HIV and HSV-2 and sexual behaviour in rural South Africa: cluster randomised controlled trial. BMJ 2008; 337: a506.
8. Gupta J, Falb KL, Lehmann H, et al. Gender norms and economic empowerment intervention to reduce intimate partner violence against women in rural Cote d'Ivoire: a randomized controlled pilot study. BMC Int Health Hum Rights 2013; 13: 46.
9. Abramsky T, Devries K, Kiss L, et al. Findings from the SASA! Study: a cluster randomized controlled trial to assess the impact of a community mobilization intervention to prevent violence against women and reduce HIV risk in Kampala, Uganda. BMC Medicine 2014; 12: 122.
10. Heise L. Violence against women: an integrated ecological framework. Violence Against Women 1998; 4: 262–90.
11. Verma R, Pulerwitz J, Mahendra vs. Promoting gender equity as a strategy to reduce HIV risk and gender-based violence among young men in India. Final Report. Washington DC: Population Council, 2008.
12. Global and regional estimates of violence against women: prevalence and health effects of intimate partner violence and non-partner sexual violence. World Health Organisation 2013.
13. The global prevalence of intimate partner homicide; a systematic review. Heidi Stöckl, Karen Devries, Alexandra Rotstein, Naeemah Abrahams, Jacquelyn Campbell, Charlotte Watts, Claudia Garcia Moreno.
14. Expert meeting on health-sector responses to violence against women, 17–19 March 2009, Geneva, Switzerland.
15. UNFPA-WAVE, Strengthening Health System Responses to Gender-based Violence in Eastern Europe and Central Asia: A resource package, 2014.
    How can health systems contribute to making gender-based violence a public health concern?

Role of Police Official in Curbing the Crime Against Women

Meeran Borwankar

Abstract

Curbing crime against women is the joint responsibility of families, community, educational institutions, workplaces and police. Role of police is to prevent such crime by effectively implementing different laws with some having been redefined and expanded recently. It can also reduce crime against women by good investigation and securing conviction of those who violate women and their rights. The article cites a few cases to substantiate author's contention of this being an issue involving society at large. It mentions need for better police population ratio, induction of more women in police, speedy trials, and witnesses joining investigation and supporting prosecution as some of the measures to reduce crime against women.

Introduction

It is surprising that most of the time citizens hold police directly responsible for crime against women. I wonder if it is because of a tendency to avoid one's own responsibility and hold someone else accountable, and in this instance men and women in 'Khaki'. While I shall talk of the role of police in detail in the article, I would first like to establish that it is the society at large and mainly the family, educational institutes and work-places that have failed to inculcate two very important lessons in the lives of citizens, first, respect for girls and women and second, equality of genders. This subsequently leads to crime against women which may be in the form of an unwanted, annoying gesture to as serious as throwing acid, a murder for dowry or a rape. I would thus open my case with the statement that it is the society, family, educational and work-places that have failed the women and need to change the environment that is biased against girl child.

Role of Police

Coming to the role of police in curbing crime against women, there are three aspects; first is the prevention, followed by investigation and then successful prosecution of offenders. For this I would argue that police is mainly responsible for curbing crime against girls and women if and when they take place in public places, e.g. teasing of women on streets, roads, market places, etc. We as police officers are aware of this issue and 'plain clothes staff' is deployed whenever there are complaints of such nature.

These 'Road Romeos' are booked under various sections of the Indian Penal Code or through State Specific Acts. It is highly recommended that girls and women approach nearest police stations or principals of schools, colleges, officials of private and public sector regularly in liaison with their local police stations or 'Chowkies' if their female students/employees are harassed at bus stops or in local trains. Silence is not an option. In fact, many young girls suffer silently and are not aware that their administrative authorities can help in curbing such cases. The key is in sustained coordination with local police officials.

The girls and women are not safe in India comes out very strongly in a survey carried out by IDFC institute during 2016–2017 at four metropolitan towns of India (Mumbai, Chennai, Bengaluru and Delhi). The survey highlighted that post 9 pm, 87% of people in Delhi started worrying about a female household member who was outside home unaccompanied. The percentages were lower in Bengaluru (54%), Chennai (48%), and Mumbai (30%). By 11 pm the percentages spiked to 97% in Delhi, 89% in Bengaluru, 90% in Chennai, and 76% in Mumbai. It highlights the need for not only police but all sections of society to come together and take concrete action for safety of women in India. It will also take us out of the scourge of poverty as the International Monetary Fund (IMF) estimates that equal participation of women in the workforce will increase India's GDP by 27%.

With reference to continuous harassment and exploitation of girls and women, I would like to refer to a notorious case known as Jalgaon Sex Scandal of Maharashtra during 1994–1995 where we came across many young college going girls having been exploited by local wealthy politicians. During investigation, most of the victims admitted not having confided in either their parents or college authorities for the fear that their further education shall be stopped. Lack of communication between girls, their families and college authorities meant that they were forced into unhealthy sexual relationships for months and years till the scandal broke out and made national news with state CID (Crime), Maharashtra taking over investigation. I am citing the case to highlight the point that the first responders in case of crime against women are family or concerned institutes. Police comes into picture later as we did by investigating the group cases of Jalgaon.

Since this particular article is for 'The Federation of Obstetric and Gynaecological Societies of India', I would like to record that the medical certificates with the comment 'victim girl is habituated to sex' made the case of prosecution very weak leading to acquittals of many cases that we had investigated as part of the Jalgaon sex scandal. During the trial girls were cross examined about these particular remarks/comments of the medical officers. However, vide the Criminal Amendment Act, 2013; defence lawyers under amended Section 146 of the Indian Evidence Act are now barred from questioning victims on this particular aspect, i.e. 'previous sexual experience'.

By the Criminal Law Amendment Act, 2013 cited above it have been made an offence under Section 166(A) if a police officer fails to record a crime against women. The delinquent police officer will be imprisoned for not less than six months which may extend to two years and fine for his/her failure to take action. It has also been added that as far as possible information and statements of victim girls and women should be recorded by women police officers.

It is a bitter truth that in India getting a FIR registered is a tough task. Politicians cite low crime rate to showcase their achievement in law enforcement. This had bred a culture of not attending to the complaints of citizens, with weaker sections of society suffering the most. Police as an organization all over the country are over worked and under staffed. The Bureau of Police Research and Development in their annual report 'Data on Police Organisation' has mentioned that sanctioned police force (Civil, District Armed Reserve (DAR), Special Armed) in India is 25,95,435 out of which actual police force (Civil, DAR and Special Armed) was 20,67,270 due to large number of vacancies. The report further mentions that police per lakh population ratio (PPR) against sanctioned police is 198.65. But due to about 20% vacancies, it comes down to about 180 police officials per lakh of population. The internationally accepted norm is 220 police officials per lakh of population. This is another reason for non-registration of crime by an over worked and under staffed police in India. Amendment of 2013 is to curb this tendency on the part of police and to ensure that crime against women is registered promptly or police officials suffer the penalty of imprisonment. However, the need to fill up the existing vacancies and to increase number of police officers cannot be ignored.

The Criminal Law Amendment Act, 2013 Further Envisages Vide Newly Added Section 166(B)

"Whoever, being in charge of a hospital, public or private, whether run by the central government, the state government, local bodies, or any other person, contravenes the provisions of Section 357C of the Code of Criminal Procedure, 1973 (2 of 1974), shall be punished with imprisonment for a term which may extend to one year or with fine or with both".

Section 357C of the Code of Criminal Procedure

"All hospitals, public or private, whether run by the central government, the state government, local bodies or any other person, shall immediately, provide the first-aid or medical treatment, free of cost, to the victims of any offence covered under Sections 326A, 376, 376A, 376B, 376C, 376D or Section 376E (acid attacks and rape cases) of the Indian Penal Code, and shall immediately inform the police of such incident."

The intent of law makers is thus clearly to provide safe environment for women and to punish those who violate it. The Criminal Law Amendment Act, 2013 and 2018 have added to the types of criminal offences against women and increased punishment especially if the victims are minor or it is a case of gang rape or by a repeat offender or the victim is in custody/charge of an authority. These amendments have introduced new sections or redefined and expanded the existing provisions under (354 and 376) in the Indian Penal Code like offences of stalking, voyeurism, etc. They have also amended the Indian Evidence Act and the Criminal Procedure Code so that a female victim is not harassed during investigation or trial of cases.

Police as an organization has taken note of these changes and have held extensive training sessions of investigating officers to improve the quality of investigation. Since e-stalking, cyber bullying of women has increased, police officers have been trained to investigate such cybercrime with latest tools and Cyber Police Stations and cells have been created. Local police station officers frequently address schools and colleges to sensitise students especially girls on safe use of cyber space to prevent crime.

Most districts in India have special units to deal with cases of domestic violence. However, as a police officer, I have been against 'all women police stations' for two reasons, one it shows distrust in the ability of men, second a woman victim must get help from the nearest police station and not be advised to go to an 'all women police station' that may be at a distance of 15–30 km. Most states having gone in for reservation for women in police, their number is gradually increasing and these inclusive police stations would prevent crime against women, investigate cases better and also provide relief to victims at the earliest. Currently the percentage of women police is 8.98% of total police in the country with Tamil Nadu having 17.46%, Bihar 15.65% and Maharashtra 12.96% women constituting their police force. Increased number of women in uniform not only deters crime against women but also signals their empowerment. It challenges the patriarchal culture of Indian society where female gender has been considered secondary to male, and is the main cause of crime against women.

There is no doubt that the Nirbhaya case (2012 Delhi gang rape and murder) and the recent Hathras gang rape case have shaken the conscience of the country and all organs of government, media and society have responded in highlighting crime against women with need for urgent change. Here it must be noted that police is a state subject and that different states have adopted different methodologies for preventing, investigating and prosecuting crime against women. Training on fresh amendments to laws and cybercrime has been imparted both by the central government through the Bureau of Police Development and Research (BPR&D), New Delhi, and also by state police training academies.

In most states Non-Governmental Organizations (NGOs) and academic institutes too are collaborating with police for prevention of crime against women and for training police personnel. After prevention and good investigation, it is successful conviction that can reduce crime against women. However, it is here that India falls short and less than 30% of cases of crime against women end in conviction. Two main reasons for the dismal performance are, very late trial of cases in courts and witnesses turning hostile by not supporting the case of prosecution. This is quite often seen in cases of domestic violence. In many cases even the victim (girl/woman) goes back on their statements. Poor investigation and prosecutors not presenting the cases in court properly also contribute to high rate of acquittal. Here I would like to mention a case of an engineering student stabbed to death by a boy, a case of one-sided love affair and a badly hurt male ego leading to the broad day light murder in Pune during 2010. Good investigation and presentation in court by the prosecutor enabled us to secure conviction in 2015, mainly because the witnesses supported prosecution despite the lag of five years in trial. Such cases need media coverage to ensure that those intending to commit crime against women are deterred.

Crime against women is rampant even at workplaces and Sexual Harassment of Women at Workplace (Prevention, Prohibition and Redressal) Act, 2013 too needs to be implemented in all seriousness it deserves. Internal Committees against such harassment are mandatory in all public and private sector offices/units. Since police has not been assigned any specific role under the Act, it emphasises the fact that community itself must take initiative to curb crime against women. Same is the case with The Protection of Women from Domestic Violence Act, 2005. It has designated 'protection officers' and police comes in picture when a cognizable offence takes place, for which as discussed above, investigating officers have been trained and their knowledge and skills updated through in-service training courses. There is definitely a strong need for more training courses for investigating officers and beat police persons for curbing and investigating crime against women.

To conclude I would say that despite sincere efforts to curb crime against women by police, India has not been successful. It highlights the need for a joint effort by family, community, educational institutes, workplaces and law enforcement agencies. To expect that police alone shall be able to curb crime against women is living in fool's paradise. Let's join hands to do our bit as doctors, teachers, industrialists, civil servants, media persons to provide safe, healthy and stimulating environment for women. And then expect and enable law enforcement agencies to come down heavily on those who do not. Amen!

SOURCE REFERENCES AND SUGGESTED READING

1. Crime Victimisation Survey IDFC Institute
2. https://in.one.un.org/unibf/gender-equality/
3. The Bureau of Police Research and Development (BPR&D) `Data on Police Organizations' 2019
4. https://bprd.nic.in/WriteReadData/userfiles/file/202001301028101694907BPRDDData2019-19forweb-2.pdf.
5. 'Crime In India' National Crime Records Bureau (NCRB).

Role of a Psychiatrist in Violence Against Women

Milan Balakrishnan

Abstract

Violence against women is widely recognised as a public health and human rights issue. Violence against woman is an also a major mental health problem. This chapter discusses the mental health impact and common physical and psychological manifestations of the problem.

Introduction

In an Indian study, on about 10000 women, 26% reported having experienced physical violence from spouses during their lifetime.[1]

It looks at how these can be identified, diagnosed and managed by the psychiatrist. Role of psychiatrist with other services and how a risk benefits balance approach should be used for the benefit of the woman.

Violence against women is widely recognised as a violation of human rights and a public health issue. Violence against women is also a prominent public mental health problem, and mental health professionals should be identifying, preventing, and responding to violence against women more effectively. The most common forms of violence against women are domestic abuse and sexual violence, and victimisation is associated with an increased risk of mental disorder.

Psychiatrists can play a key role in detecting signs of abuse, determining the level of danger, helping the individual to create a safety plan, making appropriate referrals, providing empathetic and emotional support, and providing short- and long-term trauma interventions.

Gender-based violence or violence against women is a complex social rather than biomedical problem, and addressing it means asking medical professionals to step beyond the traditional medical paradigm and work in partnership with community organizations dedicated to end this violence.

In a survey, 40% of the survivors had poor mental health.[2] Violence leads to mental disorders such as depression, post-traumatic stress disorder (PTSD), anxiety disorders, self-harm and sleep disorders.[3] Chronic violence of increased severity is associated with severe depressive disorders. In a study of female psychiatric outpatients with history of intimate partner violence, 14% were identified as having PTSD. In another study on urban women, 22.3% of them had suicidal thoughts and 3.4% had attempted suicide.[4]

Common Medical/Surgical Presentations of Violence

- Digestive problems
- Sexual dysfunction
- Hypertension
- Chronic pain
- Asthma
- Vaginal infections
- STDs
- Urinary problems
- Vaginal infections
- Pregnancy complications
- Insomnia
- Autoimmune disorders
- Fainting
- Cervical cancer

Common Psychiatric Presentations

- Alcohol abuse/dependence
- Depression
- Substance abuse
- Post-traumatic stress disorder
- Suicidality
- Anxiety
- Panic disorder

The patient may not disclose gender-based violence to you immediately. Always be aware of violence as a potential problem and develop a therapeutic relationship with the patient so she will be comfortable enough to reveal what is going on. Do not direct the patient what to do. Some individuals experiencing violence may not be yet ready to act.

Common barriers to disclosure especially in psychiatric settings is fear of consequences (e.g. the involvement of social services and child protection services), fear that disclosure will not be believed, and fear that the disclosure will lead to further violence.

Psychiatrists must be aware of these barriers and should be skilful in eliciting information. For example, in a psychiatric crisis, it is typical to use a family member to provide collateral information. "First ascertain whether the informant is an abusive partner," obtaining information from abusers can be "dangerous."

There are some critical steps to take once your patient has confirmed that some type of abuse is taking place:[5]

- Assess the level of imminent danger, which could include homicidal or suicidal threats from the partner or perpetrator, the presence of potential weapons in the home, excessive substance use, escalating verbal abuse or threats, physical or verbal abuse of children.

- Conduct this assessment in a private confidential space
- Conduct suicidal risk assessment
- Explain to the patient in detail what is going to happen so they can be less anxious, fearful and feel safe.
- The danger assessment tool can be used which assesses risk of death due to violence.
- Be non-judgemental and supportive and validate what the woman is saying
- Providing practical care and support, which responds to her concerns, but does not intrude on her autonomy.
- Listening without pressuring her to respond or disclose information
- Provide information about local community resources. These include domestic violence prevention programs, NGOs, contact numbers, mental health centres, specialized therapists, and women's shelters. It may be too dangerous for the abused person to take a pamphlet home because it can increase the danger if the perpetrator finds it. There are creative ways to provide this information—for example, a tiny piece of paper with a number can be slipped into a bag, or a pillbox.
- If the danger is imminent, have the patient call an organisation or social service while she is in your office.
- Help the patient to create an escape plan. This includes deciding where to go if she immediately needs to leave the abusive partner and packing a bag with belongings, including identification, important documents, medications if relevant, keys, phone numbers, and clothing.
- Any intervention must be guided by the principal to "do no harm", ensuring the balance between benefits and harms, and prioritizing the safety of women and their children as the uppermost concern.
- The privacy and confidentiality of the consultation, including discussing relevant documentation in the medical record and the limits of confidentiality with women, should be a priority. Therefore, good communication skills are essential.

Health care providers should discuss options and support women in their decision-making. The relationship should be supportive and collaborative, while respecting women's autonomy. Health care providers should work with the women, presenting options and possibilities, as well as providing information, with the aim to develop an effective plan and set realistic goals, but the woman should always be the one to make the decisions. In some settings, such as emergency care departments, as much as possible should be done during first contact, in case the woman does not return. Follow-up support, care, and the negotiation of safe and accessible means for follow-up consultation should be offered.

Health care providers need to have an understanding of the gender-based nature of violence against women, and of the human rights dimension of the problem. Women who have physical or mental disabilities are at an increased risk of intimate partner and sexual violence.[6,7] Health care providers should pay particular attention to their multiple needs.

Mental Health Conditions Associated with Violence Against Women

- Symptoms of depression, anxiety, PTSD, sleep disorders
- Suicidality or self-harm
- Alcohol and other substance use
- Unexplained chronic gastrointestinal symptoms
- Unexplained reproductive symptoms, including pelvic pain, sexual dysfunction
- Chronic pain (unexplained)
- Problems with the central nervous system—headaches, cognitive problems, hearing loss
- Repeated health consultations with no clear diagnosis
- There is strong evidence of an association between gender-based violence and mental health disorders among women. Women with mental health symptoms or disorders (depression, anxiety, PTSD, self-harm/suicide attempts) could be asked about gender-based violence as part of good clinical practice, particularly as this may affect their treatment and care.
- Therapeutic interventions

Brief, Structured, Psychological Treatment

Interpersonal therapy and cognitive behavioural therapy (CBT) including behavioural activation, and problem-solving treatment should be considered as psychological treatment of depressive episode/disorder in non-specialized health care settings if there are sufficient human resources (e.g. supervised community health workers). In moderate and severe depression, problem-solving treatment should be considered as adjunct treatment to pharmacological treatment.

A problem-solving approach should be considered in people with depressive symptoms (in the absence of depressive episode/disorder) that are in distress or have some degree of impaired in functioning.

Psychological treatment based on CBT principles should be considered in repeat adult help seekers with medically unexplained somatic complaints who are in substantial distress and who do not meet criteria for depressive episode.

Role of Antidepressants and Benzodiazepines

Antidepressants should not be considered for the initial treatment of adults with mild depressive episode. Tricyclic antidepressants or fluoxetine should be considered in adults with moderate to severe depressive episode/disorder.

Neither antidepressants nor benzodiazepines should be used for the initial treatment of individuals with complaints of depressive symptoms in the absence of current/prior depressive episode/disorder.

Antidepressant treatment should not be stopped before 9–12 months after recovery.

Relaxation Training and Physical Activity

Relaxation training and advice on physical activity may be considered as treatment of adults with depressive episode/disorder. In moderate and severe depression, these interventions should be considered as adjunct treatment.

Psychological Support after Recent Traumatic Event

Providing access to support based on the principles of psychological first aid should be considered for people in acute distress exposed recently to a traumatic event.

Psychological debriefing should not be used for recent traumatic event to reduce the risk of post-traumatic stress, anxiety, or depressive symptoms.

Graded self-exposure based on CBT principles in adults with post-traumatic stress disorder (PTSD) symptoms:

- If it is possible to continue to follow-up with the patient, graded self-exposure based on the principles of CBT should be considered in adults with PTSD symptoms.
- Psychological treatment based on CBT principles should be considered as treatment of people concerned about prior panic attack.
- Cognitive behavioural therapy (CBT) or eye movement desensitization and reprocessing (EMDR) interventions, delivered by health care professionals with a good understanding of violence against women, are recommended for women who are no longer experiencing violence but are suffering from PTSD.

Where children are exposed to intimate partner violence, a psychotherapeutic intervention, including sessions where they are with, and sessions where they are without their mother, should be offered.

Interventions up to 3 Months Post-trauma

Continue to offer support and care in the form of psychological first aid.

Unless the person is depressed, has alcohol or drug use problems, psychotic symptoms, is suicidal or self-harming or has difficulties functioning in day-to-day tasks, apply "watchful waiting" for 1–3 months after the event. Watchful waiting involves explaining to the woman that she is likely to improve over time and offering the option to come back for further support by making regular follow-up appointments.

If the person is incapacitated by the post-trauma symptoms (i.e. she cannot function on a day-to-day basis), arrange for cognitive behaviour therapy (CBT) or eye movement and desensitization and reprocessing (EMDR), by a health care provider with a good understanding of sexual violence.

If the person has any other mental health problems (symptoms of depression, alcohol or drug use problems, suicide or self-harm) provide care in accordance with treatment guidelines.

Interventions from 3 Months Post-trauma

Assess for mental health problems (symptoms of acute stress/PTSD, depression, alcohol and drug use problems, suicidality or self-harm) and treat depression, alcohol use disorder and other mental health disorders using guidelines

If the person has been assessed as experiencing post-traumatic stress disorder (PTSD), arrange for PTSD treatment with cognitive behaviour therapy or eye movement and desensitization reprocessing.

Consider the potential harms of psychotherapy (including CBT) when not administered properly to potentially vulnerable survivors. Informed consent and attention to safety is essential. A trained health care provider with a good understanding of sexual violence should implement therapy.

Mental Health of Perpetrators

Mental health risk factors for committing violence are:
- Alcohol and substance use disorders
- PTSD, bipolar disorder, depression, generalized anxiety disorder
- Borderline personality disorder, antisocial personality disorder
- Impulsivity, low self-control, anger, jealousy
- Exposure to violence during childhood and adolescence

Treatment of perpetrator needs evaluation and treatment for the co-morbid mental illnesses that need to be treated aggressively and even with involuntary admission due to risk of harm to self or others.

Support safe, respectful, appropriate, gender sensitive comprehensive mental health and physical health services for girls and women across the life cycle irrespective of their economic and social status, caste, or ethnocultural background.

Mandatory reporting of violence to the police by the health care provider is not recommended. However, health care providers should offer to report the incident to the appropriate authorities (including the police) if the woman wants this, and make her aware of her rights.

Child ill-treatment and life-threatening incidents must be reported to the relevant authorities by the health care provider as it is a mandatory requirement.

Providing practical care and support, which responds to her concerns, but does not intrude on her autonomy, listening without pressuring her to respond or disclose information, offering comfort and helping to alleviate or reduce her anxiety, offering information and helping her to connect to services and social supports.

Role in Advocacy

Support programs to improve the education of practicing and training other medical practitioners to recognize and treat victims of violence.

Promote safe, respectful, non-blaming, outpatient and inpatient treatment programs for women victims of violence.

Aim to undertake research to develop and evaluate the best treatments for women who have suffered from violence, and for their children and the perpetrators.

Support women's marital, sexual and reproductive choices and ensure access to safe motherhood. Support public education and awareness campaigns that increase recognition and reduce the stigma of mental illness in girls and women.

REFERENCES

1. Kumar S, Jeyaseelan L, Suresh S, Ahuja RC. Domestic violence and its mental health correlate in Indian women. Br J Psychiatry 2005;187:62–7.
2. Chandra PS, Satyanarayana VA, Carey MP. Women reporting intimate partner violence in India: associations with PTSD and depressive symptoms. Arch Women's Ment Health 2009; 12: 203–9.

3. Vachher AS, Sharma AK. Domestic violence against women and their mental health status in a colony in Delhi. Indian J Community Med 2010; 35:403–5.
4. World Health Organization. Responding to intimate partner violence and sexual violence against women: WHO clinical and policy guidelines. Geneva: WHO;2013. Available At: http://apps.who.int/iris/bitstream/10665/85240/1/9789241548595_eng.pdf?ua=1. Accessed Feb 28, 2020-02-29.
5. Stewart DE. The international consensus statement on women's mental health and the WPA consensus statement on interpersonal violence against women. World Psychiatry 2006; 5:61-4.Available at: http://www.ncbi.nlm.nih.gov/pmc/articles/PMC1472251/pdf/wpa050061.pdf.
6. Stewart DE, Robinson GE. Violence against women. In: Oldham JM, Riba MB (eds). Review of psychiatry, Vol. 14. Washington: American Psychiatric Press, 1995:261–82.
7. Dillon G, Hussain R, Loxton D, Rahman S. Mental and physical health and intimate partner violence against women: a review of the literature. Int J Family Med 2013;2013:Epub Jan 23.

Responsibilities of Society

Preeti Deshpande, Mandakini Megh

Domestic violence is a universal problem seen across countries. United Nations has organized four world conferences on women over the decades. The 1995 Fourth World Conference on Women in Beijing marked a significant turning point for the global agenda for gender equality. The Beijing Declaration and Platform for Action was adopted unanimously in 189 countries. It has an agenda for women's empowerment and considered the key global document on gender equality. It sets strategic objectives and actions for the advancement of women in critical areas of concern such as women and poverty, training of women, health, violence against women, the girl child, human rights and media issues related to women.

The world has a long way to go still. India certainly has a very long way to go. Indian culture and mythology is filled with stories of female Goddesses and stories of Swayamvaras. But there is a difference between history, stories and reality. Let's have a reality check—India is a male dominant society. The medieval era saw a downturn in women's status in the society with customs like Sati. Widows were expected to live a life of severe austerity. The woman's life was doomed if her husband died!

The winds of change began way back in the 19th Century in the British era itself. Hindu Widows' Remarriage Act was passed in 1856. Raja Ram Mohan Roy was the "Father of Indian Renaissance". He was known for his efforts to abolish Sati, child marriage, polygamy and dowry and he demanded inheritance rights for women. In 1828 he set up the "Brahmo Samaj" a reformist movement to fight against social evils.

Though a lot has improved, we still are largely an unfair society in the practical sense. We may feel the urban population is relatively liberal but even in the urban scenario women are not empowered. The government and society at large has taken several measures to enhance the status of women in India.

LEGAL PROVISIONS FOR WOMEN IN INDIA

- The Dowry Prohibition Act, 1961
- The Child Remuneration Act, 1976
- The Child Marriage Act, 1976
- The Medical Termination of Pregnancy Act, 1971
- The National Commission for Women Act, 1990

- The Protection of Human Right Act, 1983
- Protection of Women against Domestic Violence Act, 2005
- Sexual Harassment of Women at Workplace (Prevention and Prohibition and Redressal) Act, 2013

DOMESTIC VIOLENCE

Violence against women is a serious problem in India. Overall, 30% of women age 15–49 have experienced physical violence and about 6% have experienced sexual violence. In total, 36% have experienced physical or sexual violence.

The Protection of Women from Domestic Violence Act, was introduced in 2005 for effective protection of women from any kind of violence in the family and matters connected therewith.[2]

Domestic violence has been recognized since 1983 as a criminal offence under IPC 498A. It was not until enactment of the Protection of Women from Domestic Violence Act of 2005, that civil protection was afforded to victims of domestic violence. Protection of Women from Domestic Violence Act provides a definition of domestic violence that is comprehensive and includes all forms of physical, emotional, verbal, sexual and economic violence and harassment in the form of unlawful dowry demands as a form of abuse.

The Act requires appointment of protection officers to assist victims and acknowledges the importance of collaboration between government and external organization in protecting women.

Emergency Helpline Number

The government has shown a persistent commitment towards improving the law and order and safety for women. India's all-in-one emergency helpline number was launched in February 2019 by Union Home Ministry in 16 States and Union Territories. The '112' emergency helpline number would provide immediate assistance to services like police (100), fire (101), health (108), women's safety (1090) and child protection.[5]

The National Commission for Women

The National Commission for women is a statutory body of the Government of India generally concerned with advising the government on all policy matters affecting women. It was established in 1992 under the National Commission for Women Act, 1990 (Act 20 of 1990 of Government of India).[3] The objective of the National Commission for Women is to represent the rights of women in India and to provide a voice for their issues and concerns like dowry, politics, equal representation of women in jobs and domestic violence. As per the mandate the Commission investigates all matters relating to safeguards provided for women, present reports to the central government, make recommendations to the government to safeguard conditions of women, reviews from time to time and takes up issues of violation of laws relating to women and even takes Suo Moto action.

The heads under which complaints are registered with the commission include:[5]

1. Rape/attempt to rape
2. Acid attacks
3. Sexual harassment

4. Sexual assault
5. Stalking/voyeurism
6. Trafficking/prostitution
7. Outraging the modesty of women
8. Cybercrimes against women
9. Dowry harassment
10. Dowry death
11. Bigamy/polygamy
12. Protection of women against domestic violence
13. Right to marriage by choice
14. Divorce
15. Right to live with dignity
16. Gender discrimination
17. Denial of maternity benefit
18. Indecent representation of women
19. Sex selected abortion

The National Commission analyses complaints received[4]

- This shows the trend of crimes against women and suggests system changes needed for reduction of crimes.
- The complaints are analyzed to understand gaps in the routine functioning of the government in tackling violence against women and corrective measures are suggested.
- The complaints are also used as case studies for sensitization programmes for police, judiciary, prosecutors, forensic scientists, lawyers and administrative functionaries.

The commission helps in processing complaints on Acts related to justice for women. The complaints are processed in the following manner[4]

- Investigations by police are expedited and monitored
- Family disputes are resolved through counselling or hearing before the commission.
- For serious crimes, the commission constitutes an inquiry committee which makes spot enquiries, examines witnesses, collects evidences and submits the report with recommendations. Such investigations provide immediate relief and justice to the victims of violence and atrocities. The implementation of the report is monitored by the National Commission for Women. There is a provision for having experts/lawyers on these committees.
- A few complaints are also forwarded to the respective State Commission for Women and other forums like National Human Rights Commission, National Commission for Scheduled Caste and Scheduled Tribes.

As per the mandate, the commission also undertakes special studies, organizes seminars, conferences and workshops in collaboration with NGOs, voluntary organizations and colleges. It also organizes programmes like Violence Free Homes—a joint programme held by National Commission for Women, Delhi Police and TISS, Mumbai.

The commission also participates in planning socio-economic development of women and works on women's empowerment.

As per the **National Family Health Survey 4**, it was found that in families approximately 30% of women were employed compared to 97% of men who were employed. Also it was found that amongst working women 50% earn less than the husband. Even where women are working, it was found in 15% husband decides how the cash will be spent and 60% both decide. But regarding the husband's earnings 25–30% husbands will decide how the cash will be spent. Only about 8–10% women are empowered to make choices about their own health. Also the women are not empowered to fend for themselves as they are not empowered to move out of their homes alone much (only 30–40%) till the age of 25 years. However, amongst older women 45–70% are allowed to fend for themselves.[1]

So, as per the survey women are as yet poorly empowered. Women's empowerment can help in countering issues of domestic violence.

12% of married women with 12 or more years of education have experienced spousal violence, compared with 21% of married women whose husbands have 12 or more years of education. This suggests that women's own education reduces their likelihood of experiencing spousal violence more than their husband's education.

Spousal violence is lower among couples in which husbands and wives have both been to school and are equally educated (24%) than among couples where the husband has more education than the wife or if neither husband nor wife are educated (46%).[1]

Sexual Harassment in Workplace Act, 2013

- Sexual Harassment of Women at Workplace (Prevention and Prohibition and Redressal) Act, 2013 was passed which is consistent with the Vishakha Guidelines.
- The Vishakha Guidelines placed responsibility on the employer to ensure that all women did not face a hostile environment at the workplace. However, there was no punishment in place if the guidelines were not followed. Hence, the Act was needed.
- As per the guidelines, a complaints committee should be headed by a woman employees, at least 50% of the members should be women and a third party like NGOs should be involved. The guideline covered paid, voluntary, public and private sectors.
- As per the guideline it is obligatory for the employer to ensure equality and dignity at workplace
- The Act provides civil remedy to women
- An internal complaints committee is mandatory for any workplace with 10 or more employees.
- If the workplace has less than 10 employees or if the complaint is against the employer himself the complainant can go to a local complaints committee at the district level.

Women's Reservation Bill

- Women's Reservation Bill was initially introduced in the Parliament in September 1996. The bill was introduced in Lok Sabha by the United Front Government.
- The main aim of the bill was to reserve 33% of the seats in Lok Sabha and all State Legislative Assemblies for women.

- Reservation criteria: As per the bill, the seats will be reserved on a rotational basis. The seats would be determined by a draw of lots in such a way that a seat would only be reserved once in every 3 consecutive general election.
- Vajpayee government pushed for the bill in Lok Sabha but it still was not passed.
- UPA-1 government, led by Congress, again introduced the bill to reserve seats for women in Lok Sabha and legislative assemblies in May 2008.
- After its reintroduction, the bill was passed by Rajya Sabha on March 2010, but was still left pending in the Lok Sabha.

Women actually form 48% of the population. It is a very fair bill for adequate representation of women in the government. Unfortunately the bill has yet not been passed.

Most Women do not Seek Help when they are Abused

Only one in four abused women have ever sought help to try to end the violence they have experienced. Two out of three women have not only never sought help, but have also never told anyone about the violence. Abused women most often seek help from their own families (65%). The second most common source of help is the husband's family (29%). 15% sought help from a friend. Only 3% sought help from the police. 2% sought help from religious leaders. About 1% seek help from doctors or medical personnel.

Our Role as Medical Professionals

The first and foremost responsibility of medical institutions is that they cannot refuse treatment to the aggrieved woman under any circumstances. Detection of injuries arising from domestic violence and identification of "Domestic violence as a syndrome" is a concept somewhat similar to "Battered baby syndrome". If identified the person in-charge will be required to counsel the woman in privacy and inform her about the reliefs under this law.

The treatment and documentation should be done with gendered understanding in view. Also referrals to other related services such as counselling and legal aid is a part of the duty of the medical professionals. Hospitals may have to function as temporary shelter homes. Domestic violence is to be recognized as a medical emergency (Figure 15.1).

Role of Service Providers and Non-Governmental Organisations

Many Non-Governmental Organisations have taken up issues of gender-based violence. They are involved in providing support, shelter homes, rehabilitation and empowerment of victims of domestic violence. They are also involved in running social and community awareness and sensitization programmes.

One such organization is the Family Planning Association of India established since 1949. It works closely with NGOs and the government. It is the founding member of the International Planned Parenthood Federation. It has taken up issues of gender-based violence, i.e. violence against an individual based on his biological sex or gender identity. Gender-based violence includes physical violence, sexual, verbal, emotional and psychological abuse, also coercion, economic and educational deprivation.

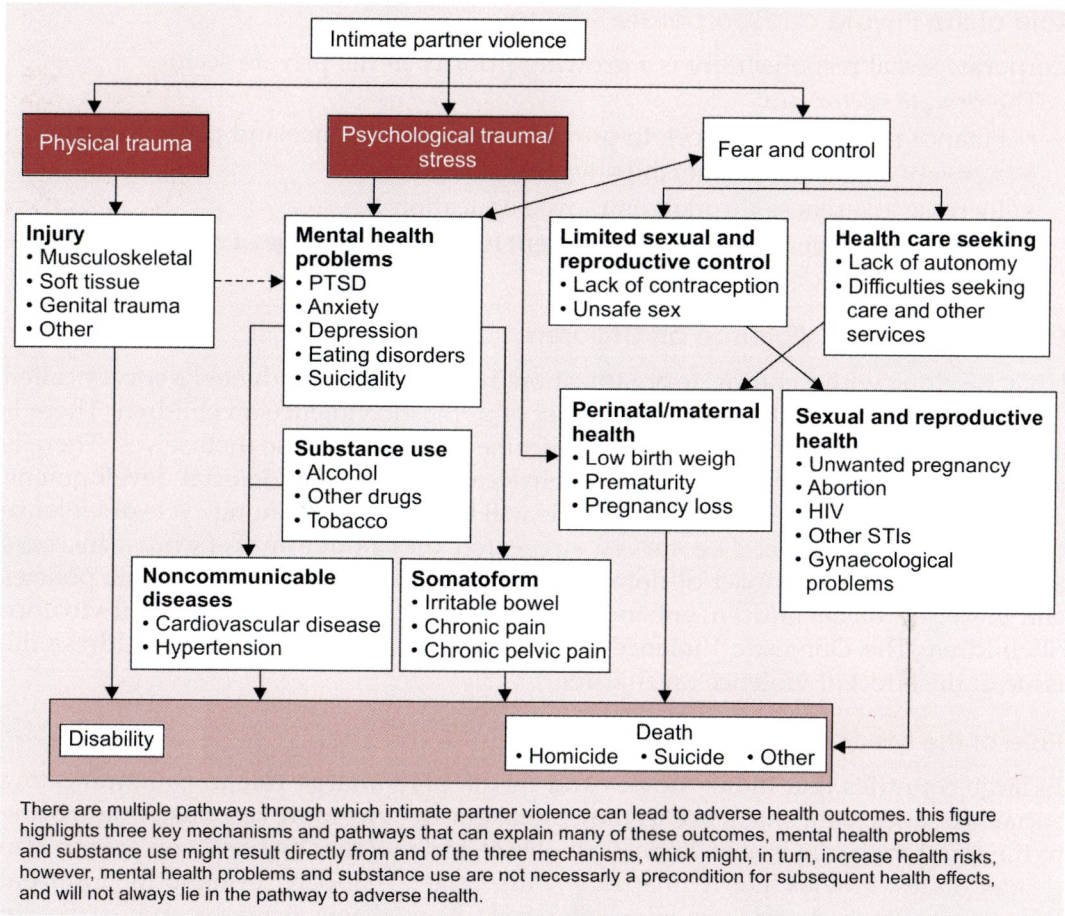

There are multiple pathways through which intimate partner violence can lead to adverse health outcomes. this figure highlights three key mechanisms and pathways that can explain many of these outcomes, mental health problems and substance use might result directly from and of the three mechanisms, whick might, in turn, increase health risks, however, mental health problems and substance use are not necessarily a precondition for subsequent health effects, and will not always lie in the pathway to adverse health.

Figure 15.1: Pathways and health effects of intimate partner violence[7]

Impact of Domestic Violence is at Multiple Levels

Domestic violence has an impact on the women's health. As per the WHO, these women are twice as likely to experience depression, anorexia or alcohol disorders. They are 16% more likely to have low birth weight babies and 1.5 times more likely to get HIV and sexually transmitted diseases. Domestic violence increases chances of injuries and premature death. Also there is a higher chance of unwanted pregnancies, anaemia and chronic ill health. Various programmes are run by NGOs, National Women's Commission and Medical Organizations to create awareness and change the outlook of the society. *Stree Hinsa Mukt*.

Bharat Abhiyan is one such programme run by the Family Planning Association of India with an objective to catalyze the civil society for preventing and mitigating violence against women. It includes encouraging the society to take a pledge to denounce violence. Doctors involved in this programme have to identify the history of domestic violence and provide treatment, counselling and referrals. It involves empowering young women with life skills and training. It also entails enabling men and boys to break away from the rigid norms of patriarchy.

Role of the Private and Corporate Sectors

Corporate social responsibility is a growing priority in the private sector.

The private sector can:
- Finance initiatives that seek to prevent domestic violence and protect victims
- Actively engage in partnerships with NGOs
- Increase awareness through employee education
- Take action to persuade the government to take up the issue of domestic violence and its impact on children seriously.

Effect of Domestic Violence on Children

UNICEF along with a corporate organization the body shop conducted a survey called "Behind closed doors" to study the impact of domestic violence on children. There is an increased risk that the children may become victims of abuse themselves. There is a significant risk of harm to the child's physical, emotional and social development. There is a strong social likelihood that this will become a continuing cycle of violence for the next generation. The survey suggested that policy makers must increase awareness about the impact of domestic violence on children, create public policies and laws to protect children, enhance social services that address impact of violence of children. The Domestic Violence Act currently does not specifically address the issue of the effect of violence on children.[8]

Role of the Media

In large countries like India, movies and media play a large role in communicating social messages to the masses. Our movie-makers are now more responsible and bring to the forefront social issues domestic violence and violence against women and also gender biases. Movies like "Chhapak", "Pink" and "Thappad" bring to the forefront the stigma attached to the women who fight back. Their struggles may strike an empathic chord with many sufferers, their family and friends.

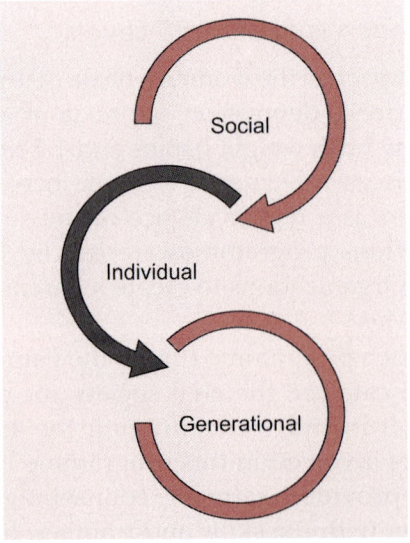

Figure 15.2: Impact of domestic violence

The role of news reporting media cannot be refuted in case such as the Jessica Lal murder case where the perpetrator was brought to book only because of media support.

The advertising media is also an indicator of how women are being portrayed. The International Advertising Association, Indian Chapter, in association with Hansa Research and supported by UNFPA and Ladli NGO did a survey on 'the portrayal of women in advertising' across senior advertising and marketing professionals—Is it in sync with their status in society? Has there been a change for the better?

Advertising is the torch bearer of change in the society. Women are now being shown as multi-taskers and individualistic. Women must not be stereotyped, objectified and commodified. Women are now viewed as potential consumers as they have education and financial independence (Figure 15.2).

CONCLUSION

In social-cultural level, to bring the idea of gender equality to public is one tough mission for the government. The process of social change is obscure however the effects are obvious. Only in a more gender-equal society, women who have suffered violence could get rid of shame/self-blame and such happenings could be de-stigmatized. Family, school, peer groups, and media are all agencies of social change, which all together should join the cultural revolution and mental revolution to construct India into a more female-friendly society. Domestic violence concerns so many elements. Low rates of participation in education, lack of economic independence, value biases operating against women, etc. directly and indirectly resulted in the women been given the status of being the secondary gender in Indian society.

The winds of change need to gain momentum. I would like to end with the quote of the famous philosopher Augustine of Hippo:

Right is right even if no one is doing it;
Wrong is wrong even if everyone is doing it.

REFERENCES

1. National Family Healthy Survey-4 (NFHS-4)-2015-2016-International Institute for Population Sciences, Deonar, Mumbai 400008, Ministry of Health and Family Welfare.
2. Protection of Women from Domestic Violence Act, 2005 published by Ministry of Law and Justice.
3. National Commission for Women http://ncw.nic.in/commission/about-us.
4. National Commission for Women http://ncw.nic.in/ncw-cells/complaint-investigation-cell.
5. 112 is India's all-in-one-emergency helpline number. http://www.inidatoday.in/information.in/information/story/112-inida's-all-in-one-emergency-helpline-number-kow-all-about-it-1461757-2019-02021.
6. Stree Hinsa Mukt Bharat Abhiyan, FPA, India.
7. Global and Regional estimates of violence against women: prevalence and health effects of intimate partner violence and non-partner sexual violence, World Health Organisation 2013.
8. Behind Closed Doors: The Impact of Domestic Violence on Children, Survery by UNICEF with the Body Shop.

Implementing a Comprehensive Health Care Response to Sexual Violence

Sangeeta Rege, Padma Bhate-Deosthali, Sanjida Arora

The chapter seeks to present legal responsibilities of health care providers (HCPs) in responding to sexual violence along with key highlights related to POCSO and Criminal Amendment to Rape. While doing so, we aim to dispel notions about rape using research evidence and provide a framework for implementation of comprehensive health care to survivors of sexual violence.

Background

The health systems and health professionals play a crucial role in responding to survivors of sexual violence. They have therapeutic as well as forensic roles mandated by laws on sexual violence. Both the POCSO 2012 (Protection of Children from Sexual Offences Act, 2012) and CLA 2013 (Criminal Law Amendment Act, 2013) recognise the need for immediate care for survivors of sexual violence over and above the medico-legal role of doctors. These changes were spurred by the massive campaign following the brutal gang rape of a young woman in Delhi which stirred the nation in December 2012. It brought forth concerns related to gaps in state response to sexual violence. Archaic definition of rape, procedural failures in investigations, inadequacies in medico-legal response by the health sector and institutional biases amongst others received attention of the media and society at large.

It is in this context that the Ministry of Health and Family Welfare, Union of India (MoHFW, 2014) responded and developed procedural guidelines along with a protocol for medical professionals to respond to survivors/victims of sexual violence in 2014. The protocol enables providers to respond to the issue of sexual violence in a gender sensitive and scientific manner. It recommended discarding the two-finger test and reiterated that comments on "habituation to sexual activity" should be forbidden from the medical examination reports. Medical providers were advised to document only signs of fresh injury to the hymen.

Defining Sexual Violence

WHO defines sexual violence as: "Any sexual Act, attempt to obtain a sexual Act, unwanted sexual comments or advances, or Acts to traffic women's sexuality, using coercion, threats of harm or physical force, by any person regardless of relationship to the victim, in any setting, including but not limited to home and work." The focus is on the term "non-consensual": An Act cannot be considered consensual if consent is offered, under threat/under false agreement/or person is unable to give consent due to unsoundness of mind.

In India, the definition of rape was broadened through two important laws; POCSO 2012 and Criminal Law Amendment Act, 2013. It expanded the definition of rape to include oral/urethral/anal penetration, use of fingering and use of objects (other than penis) for vaginal, urethral and anal penetration. The expanded scope to also bring in manipulation of any part of the body of a child/woman so as to cause penetration into the vagina, urethra, anus or any other part of body. As far as POCSO 2012 is considered, definition of sexual violence also includes sexual harassment of children defined as by use of any words/gestures/sounds with sexual intent to a child or exhibitionism of body part, use of children for pornography amongst others. While the changes in law are welcome and most needed, the law related to rape of adults does not consider rape of marginalised sections of the community such as intersex persons and transgender persons. Similarly, the rape law in India does not recognise rape by a husband on his wife. There is an urgent need to expand the scope of the law and include these aspects.

Legal Obligation of Health Facilities

The legal changes related to definition of rape have several implications on medical evidence as the nature of sexual violence and circumstances of the assault determine the kind of medical evidence that may or may not be found on the body of the survivor. Additional progressive amendments were also made in the law including recording the offence of rape in a place where survivor is comfortable, recording Section 164 CrPC statement of a survivor in front of judicial magistrate, explicit enlisting of duties of medical providers, special provisions for in camera trials, directions for women judges to preside in hearings as far as practicable and compensation by states to survivors were also changes in the law.

An important change in the law is also inclusion of Section 357C, which indicates that all hospitals run by public or private, whether run by central government, state government, local bodies or any person, shall immediately provide the first aid, or medical treatment, free of cost and inform the police of such incident. An important provision that concerns the medical providers is Section 166B. The section states that whoever is in-charge of a hospital, public or private, whether run by central government, state government, local bodies or any person, if does not provide immediate medico-legal care shall be imprisoned for 1 year or be fined or both.

Components of a comprehensive health care response to sexual assault: The model comprises the following aspects:

- Operationalising informed consent for survivors of sexual violence
- Carrying out systematic documentation of history of sexual violence
- Using gender sensitive protocols for examination and collection of relevant forensic evidence
- Recording a reasoned medical opinion
- Providing first contact psychological support and free medical support
- Maintaining a clear and fool-proof chain of custody.

CEHAT actively paved the way towards establishing right to health care for survivors through its work involving direct intervention with survivors, training of health care providers, research and legal advocacy since 2008. This was much before the changes in law. It set a comprehensive model in three hospitals in collaboration with the MCGM. Such a response was an extension of efforts of MCGM to respond to VAW. One of the first efforts by the corporation was made in 2000, in collaboration with CEHAT to set up a hospital-based crisis centre called Dilaasa*. At Dilaasa, hospital staff were equipped to recognize VAW as a public health issue, and identify violence amongst patients coming to the hospital as part of clinical enquiry. CEHAT has also engaged with the authors of Modi's Textbook on Medical Jurisprudence and Toxicology prominent book on forensic medicine; got to its latest edition replace the chapter related to rape examination and drew it majorly from protocol and guidelines for medico-legal examination of rape by MoHFW (Kannan, 2016). This change was significant because courts heavily relied on Modi's medical jurisprudence while deciding upon rape trials.

Health Consequences of Rape

Physical	Psychological
• Injuries • Sexually transmitted infections • HIV • Unwanted pregnancy • Pelvic inflammatory disease • Urinary tract infections • Genital fistulae	• Loss of power because rape is experienced as an episode of overwhelming powerlessness • Fear of another episode/fear of threat to life • Loss of trust • Feelings of being dirtied and loss of self-worth • Desire to avoid social contact • Fear of sexual contact • Nightmares and flash backs • Feelings of shame, embarrassment • Suicide ideation

Role of Examining Doctor: A doctor has both therapeutic role that comprises providing medical treatment and psychological care as well as a forensic role that comprises conducting medico-legal examination, collection of evidence and provide a reasonable medical opinion. A few aspects that need to be kept in mind are:

1. **Informed written consent by medical provider should be sought specifically for**
   - Medical examination and treatment for consequences of sexual violence
   - With a police requisition after making a police complaint
   - With a court directive

   Informed consent should also enable survivor to withdraw her consent if she feels that she does not want to go ahead with examination and evidence collection. In such instances a medical provider must explain benefits and consequences of undergoing examination, but the final word would be that of the survivor. In such instances it should be recorded on the hospital records along with a signature of the survivor.

   Survivors above 12 years (Section 89 of IPC) of age can give consent for treatment. If a survivor is below 12 years or incapacitated/unsound, then parental/guardian consent should be sought. In the absence of guardian-consent can be sought from

---

*Dilaasa is India's 1st hospital based crisis centre. It is a joint initiative of MCGM and CEHAT. It has now been replicated in several states of India and has been financially supported by NUHM.

senior medical officer in case of an unaccompanied minor survivor as per hospital policy. The consent form should be signed by the survivor and the doctor.

2. **Seeking history of sexual violence:** The first step is to establish rapport so that survivor feels safe and hence key principles to be implemented in it as ensuring a nonjudgmental attitude and a nonthreatening environment. All efforts should be made to ensure privacy. A detailed history seeking can enable examination procedure and guides evidence collection. Health care providers (HCPs) also need to understand that there are different forms of rape that occur and hence they need to develop a language as well as be comfortable to explore oral anal and vaginal nonconsensual Acts. The details of rape should be recorded verbatim as it has evidentiary value.

3. **Asking for relevant medical history:** Relevant surgical and medical history is important in the medico-legal care for rap survivors. Important aspects such as onset of menarche, whether menstruation occurred at the time of incident, last menstrual period should be sought. History of menstruation is sought to understand that evidence can be lost with menstrual blood and may require re-examination in order to visualize injuries if any. It is however advised that aspects like height-weight, GPLAD should not be recorded as they have no relevance to sexual violence being examined and treated and in fact lead to casting aspersions on the gynaecological and sexual history of a survivor of rape.

4. **Details of the sexual assault history to be sought:** A doctor should note date of incident being reported to the hospital, whether it was a single episode or multiple incidents, if the survivor recalls the number of assailants and names if known. Description of the episode should be in the words of the survivor—this has legal relevance. Besides sexual violence, doctor can also seek information on types of physical violence, emotional violence, verbal threats or whether survivor was given or alcohol being given to survivor.

5. **General and genital examination:** A careful examination of both body and genitals with the objective of the examination being to look for any signs of harm, not just for injuries. An important aspect to be remembered is that while recording injures only fresh record that which is relevant to the assault—for instance old tears and tags to hymen should not be recorded as they serve no purpose and in fact are damaging as such documentation lends itself to character assassination. Hence, only fresh tear, edema to the hymen and fresh bleeding should be recorded. Another aspect to be kept in mind that size of vaginal introitus should not be recorded—it is akin to 'two-finger test' which has been barred by Supreme Court. All injuries can be marked on body charts as they assist in visual appreciation.

6. **Examination for determining medical age:** There are a lot of misconceptions related to ways of carrying out age estimation. However, it should be carried out only if a survivor does not have any document stating her age. Scientific method of age estimation is to carry out examination based on physical growth, dental analysis and radiological findings. The practitioner should create a mean of the three tests.

7. **Treatment and care:** Some important aspects to be remembered are:
   • Psychological first aid
   • STI prevention treatment

- Emergency contraception
- Wound treatment
- Tetanus prophylaxis
- Hepatitis B vaccination
- Postexposure prophylaxis for HIV

8. **Evidence collection:** One of the most important aspects to remember in medico-legal examination is the scope and relevance of evidence collection. Only relevant evidence should be collected. Evidence collection has a direct relationship to the nature of assault, the time lapse between the episode of sexual violence and reaching a health facility and activities leading to loss of evidence. These activities range from cleaning oneself, washing, douching, urination, defecation, gargling and bathing. It is natural for a survivor to clean herself after an assault and so she should not be admonished for it. Instead the doctor should note these activities and analyse the role they have played in loss of evidence. Examining doctor must explain the nature of sample collected for which purpose, e.g. vulval swab for presence of semen.

9. **Medical opinion:** Medical opinion forms an important aspect of medico-legal responsibilities of a health provider. Such responsibility is also vested in the doctor by the law. The law disallows medical providers from usage of the term "Rape occurred or rape did not occur" in the medical opinion as rape is a legal term. Medical opinion is an interpretation of the findings or lack of medical findings based on an immediate examination. Hence, medical opinion is divided into provisional and final opinion. The final opinion is based on the receipt of Forensic Science Laboratory (FSL) reports based on evidence sent for analysis.

Emerging Evidence from CEHAT's Engagement with Public Hospitals on Rape Response

- A total of 728 rape survivors were provided medico-legal care for rape. 67% survivors were under the ages of 18 years. There has been a 3-fold increase in reporting of rape—94 (2008–2012) to 354 in (2013–2015). 20% survivors reported on their own to hospital while 80% were brought by police to hospitals.
- In 70% cases the perpetrators were known to survivors of 728 rape survivors, 15 were boys and 2 were transgender persons. It is important to recognize that people form lesbian, gay, bisexual, transgender, queer and intersex (LGBTQI) communities face sexual violence. Doctors must be skilled to provide care.
- The MoHFW medico-legal protocol also enabled documentation of circumstances in which rape occurred. 23% survivors narrated that they were unable to resist the Act as they were too shocked and scared, an additional 14 and survivors stated they were restrained physically and could not resist the abuser. While 29% survivors were too small in age to resist sexual violence. A few survivors managed to scream (13%) and resisted by (10%) by fighting and pushing the abuser away.
- The medico-legal protocol analysis also helped to analyse different factors that leads to loss of forensic evidence. These are important and educative aspects for the health providers.

Challenges to Implementation of Comprehensive Health Care Response to Rape

- Mandatory reporting by hospitals of all rape has jeopardized access to health services. Consensual sex amongst persons under 18 years is also being criminalized.
- Concept of "informed refusal" by survivors who do not wish to record an FIR is a useful tool. It allows doctors to record reasons for refusal to make a police complaint. A copy of it stays with the hospital with signature of survivor.
- Documentation can help the doctors to appear in the court of law and enable them to perform their therapeutic role-offering MTP services, contraceptive advice, etc.
- Courts, police and doctors continue to essentialise presence of injuries in medical examination. It is important to dispel these notions based on evidence.
- Doctors are unable to provide a final medical opinion due to delay or non-receipt of FSL reports.
- Doctors are also not equipped to present their findings or reasons for lack of findings in the court.
- It is important to carry out an interface between doctors, police and courts for clarity on the role of doctors, its scope and limitations of medical evidence.

Annexure 1: CEHAT and MCGM, 2018

Resistance/lack of resistance	Frequency	Percent
Resisted by screaming/running away	68	13
Resisted by fighting (pushing away, scratching)	50	10
Unable to resist because physically restrained	74	14
Unable to resist because drugged/unconscious/sleeping	50	10
Unable to resist due to threats/fear	128	23
Too small to understand/resist/mentally challenged	154	29
Unconscious so history is not clear	4	1
Total	528	100

Details: It must be understood that Act of rape does not require physical force. As seen that almost 48% could not resist owing to threats/fear/being unconscious/or too small to comprehend the Act.

Post-rape Activities and Loss of Evidence

Activities leading to loss of evidence

Nature of activities	Frequency	Percent
Voided urine	406	79
Eaten food	346	66
Ingested fluid	356	68
Changed clothes	330	63
Defecated	306	56
Bathed	288	56
Douched	206	40

- Survivor's immediate reaction is to clean herself after rape as seen in activities mentioned above and this has a bearing on loss of medical evidence.

Annexure 2: Table indicative of type of evidence to be collected

History of sexual violence	Type of swab	Purpose	Points to consider
Peno-vaginal	Vaginal swabs	• Semen/sperm detection • Lubricant • DNA	• Whether ejaculation occurred inside vagina or outside • Use of condom
	Body swabs	• Semen/sperm detection • Saliva (in case of sucking/licking)	• If ejaculation occurred outside
Peno-anal	Anal swabs	• Semen/sperm detection • DNA • Lubricant • Faecal matter	• Whether ejaculation occurred inside anus or outside • Use of condom
	Body swabs	• Semen/sperm detection • Saliva (in case of sucking/licking)	• If ejaculation occurred outside
Peno-oral	Oral swabs	• Semen/sperm detection • DNA • Saliva	• Whether ejaculation occurred inside mouth or outside • Use of condom
	Body swabs	• Semen/sperm detection • Saliva (in case of sucking/licking)	• If ejaculation occurred outside
Use of objects	Swab of the orifice (anal, vaginal and/or oral)	Lubricant	Detection of lubricant used if any
Use of body parts (fingering)	Swab of the orifice (anal, vaginal and/or oral)	Lubricant	
Masturbation	Swab of the orifice/body part	• Semen/sperm detection • DNA • Lubricant	• Whether ejaculation occurred or not • If ejaculated in orifice or body parts

SOURCE REFERENCES AND SUGGESTED READING

1. Centre for Enquiry into Health and Allied Themes, Maharashtra University of Health Sciences, Directorate of Medical Education and Research. Integrating gender in medical education: forensic medicine and toxicology: a guide for medical teachers. Mumbai: Centre for Enquiry into Health and Allied Themes, Maharashtra University of Health Sciences, Directorate of Medical Education and Research; 2017.
2. Centre for Enquiry into Health and Allied Themes, Municipal Corporation of Greater Mumbai. Understanding dynamics of sexual violence: study of case records. Mumbai: Centre for Enquiry into Health and Allied Themes, Municipal Corporation of Greater Mumbai; 2018.
3. India. Criminal Law (Amendment) Act (2013). New Delhi: 2013.
4. India. Ministry of Health & Family Welfare. Guidelines & Protocols: medico-legal care for survivors/victims of sexual violence. New Delhi: Government of India; 2014.
5. India. Ministry of Women and Child Development. The Protection of Children from Sexual Offences Act (2012). New Delhi: Government of India; 2012.
6. Kannan K. Modi: A Textbook of Medical Jurisprudence and Toxicology. 25th ed. New Delhi: Lexis Nexis & Butterworths; 2016.
7. Verma JS, Seth L, Subramanian G. Justice JS Verma Committee. Report of the committee on amendments to criminal law. New Delhi: Government of India; 2013.

Section

IV

Protocols and Practical Approach to Cases

Prerequisites of Examination— Who, How, When!! and Concept of One Stop Crisis Centre

Hema Relwani

Health professionals play a dual role in responding to the survivors of sexual assault.[1]
1. To provide the required medical treatment and psychological support.
2. To assist survivors in their medico-legal proceedings by collecting evidence and ensuring a good quality documentation.

Every hospital must have a standard operating procedure (SOP) for management of cases of sexual violence:[1]
1. To provide comprehensive services.
2. For the smooth handling of the cases and clarity of roles of each staff.
3. To have uniform practice across all doctors in the hospital.

WHO[1]

- Any registered medical practitioner can conduct the examination and it is not mandatory for a gynaecologist to examine such a case.
- In case of a girl or woman, every possible effort should be made to find a female doctor but absence of availability of lady doctor, one should not deny or delay the treatment and examination.
- In case a female doctor is not available for the examination of a female survivor, a male doctor should conduct the examination in the presence of a female attendant.
- In case of a minor/person with disability, his/her parent/guardian/any other person with whom the survivor is comfortable may be present.
- In the case of a transgender/intersex person, the survivor should be given a choice as to whether she/he wants to be examined by a female doctor, or a male doctor. In case a female doctor is not available, a male doctor may conduct the examination in the presence of a female attendant.
- Police personnel must not be allowed in the examination room during the consultation with the survivor.
- If the survivor requests, her relative may be present while the examination is done. There must be no delay in conducting an examination and collecting evidence. Providing treatment and necessary medical investigations are the prime responsibility of the examining doctor. Admission, evidence collection or filing a police complaint is not mandatory for providing treatment.

WHERE[1]

The history taking and examination should be carried out in complete privacy in the special room set up in the hospital for examination of sexual violence survivor.

The room should have
- adequate space,
- sufficient lighting,
- a comfortable examination table,
- all the pieces of equipment required for a thorough examination, and
- the sexual assault forensic operational issues 20 evidence Sexual Assault Forensic Evidence (SAFE) Kit containing the following items for collecting and preserving physical evidence following a sexual violence:
  - Forms for documentation
  - Large sheet of paper to undress over
  - Paper bags for clothing collection
  - Catchment paper
  - Sterile cotton swabs and swab guards for biological evidence collection
  - Comb
  - Nail cutter
  - Wooden stick for fingernail scrapings
  - Small scissors
  - Urine sample container
  - Tubes/vials/vaccutainers for blood samples [ethylene diamine tetra-acetic acid (EDTA), plain, sodium fluoride]
  - Syringes and needle for drawing blood
  - Distilled water
  - Disposable gloves
  - Glass slides
  - Envelopes or boxes for individual evidence samples
  - Labels
  - Lac (sealing wax) stick for sealing
  - Clean clothing
  - Shower/hygiene items for survivors use after the examination

Other items for a forensic/medical examination and treatment that may be included are:[1]
- Wood's lamp/good torch
- Vaginal speculums
- Drying rack for wet swabs and/or clothing
- Patient gown, cover sheet, blanket, pillow
- Post: It notes to collect trace evidence
- Camera (35 mm, digital with colour printer)
- Microscope
- Colposcope/magnifying glass
- Toluidine blue dye
- 1% acetic acid diluted spray

- Urine pregnancy test kit
- Surgilube
- Medications

The collected samples for evidence may be preserved in the hospital till such time that police are able to complete their paper work for dispatch to forensic lab test including DNA.

After the examination is complete the survivor should be permitted to wash up, using the toiletries and the clothing provided by the hospital if her own clothing is taken as evidence.

Admission should not be insisted upon unless the survivor requires indoor stay for observation/treatment.

Survivors of sexual violence should receive all services completely free of cost. This includes OPD/inpatient registration, lab and radiology investigations, urine pregnancy test (UPT) and medicines.

The casualty medical officer must label the case papers for any sexual violence case as "free" so that free treatment is ensured. Medicines should be prescribed from those available in the hospital.

If certain investigations or medicines are not available, the social worker at the hospital should ensure that the survivor is compensated for investigations/medicines from outside.

A copy of all documentation (including that pertaining to medico-legal examination and treatment) must be provided to the survivor free of cost.

The stepwise approach to be used for a comprehensive response to the sexual violence survivor as follows:

i. Initial resuscitation/first aid
ii. Informed consent for examination, evidence collection, police procedures
iii. Detailed history taking
iv. Medical examination
v. Age estimation (physical/dental/radiological)—if requested by the investigating agency.
vi. Evidence collection as per the protocol
vii. Documentation
viii. Packing, sealing and handing over the collected evidence to police
ix. Treatment of injuries
x. Testing/prophylaxis for STIs, HIV, hepatitis B and pregnancy
xi. Psychological support and counselling
xii. Referral for further help (shelter, legal support).

DOCUMENTATION

Record the name of hospital where the survivor is being examined followed by the following:[1]

- Name, address, age and sex (male/female/other) of the survivor.
- Date and time of receiving the patient in the hospital and commencement of examination.

- Name of the person who brought the survivor and relationship to accompanying persons.
- Informed consent:
  A survivor may approach a health facility under three circumstances:
  a. on his/her own only for treatment for effects of assault;
  b. with a police requisition after police complaint; or
  c. with a court directive.
- If a person has come directly to the hospital without the police requisition, the hospital is bound to provide treatment and conduct a medical examination with consent of the survivor/parent/guardian (depending on age). A police requisition is not required for this.
- If a person has come on his/her own without FIR, he/she may or may not want to lodge a complaint but requires a medical examination and treatment. Even in such cases the doctor is bound to inform the police as per law. However, neither court nor police can force the survivor to undergo medical examination. It has to be with the informed consent of the survivor/parent/guardian (depending on the age).
- In case the survivor does not want to pursue a police case, a MLC must be made and she must be informed that she has the right to refuse to file FIR. An informed refusal must be documented in such cases.
- If the person has come with a police requisition or wishes to lodge a complaint later, the information about medico-legal case (MLC) no. and police station should be recorded.
- Doctors are legally bound to examine and provide treatment to survivors of sexual violence.
- Police personnel should not be present during any part of the examination.

Consent should be taken for the following purposes:
- Examination
- Sample collection for clinical and forensic examination, treatment
- Police intimation.

Doctors shall inform the person being examined about the nature and purpose of examination and in case of child to the child's parent/guardian/or a person in whom the child reposes trust. This information should include:

- The medico-legal examination is to assist the investigation, arrest and prosecution of those who committed the sexual offence. This may involve an examination of the mouth, breasts, vagina, anus and rectum as necessary depending on the particular circumstances.
- To assist investigation, forensic evidence may be collected with the consent of the survivor. This may include removing and isolating clothing, scalp hair, foreign substances from the body, saliva, pubic hair, samples taken from the vagina, anus, rectum, mouth and collecting a blood sample.
- The survivor or in case of child, the parent/guardian/or a person in whom the child reposes trust, has the right to refuse either a medico-legal examination or collection of evidence or both, but that refusal will not be used to deny treatment to survivor after sexual violence.
- The survivor or guardian may refuse to give consent for any part of examination, however, the refusal should be respected. It should also be explained that refusal for such examination will not affect/compromise treatment. Such informed refusal for examination and evidence collection must be documented.

- In case there is informed refusal for police intimation, then that should be documented. At the time of MLC intimation being sent to the police, a clear note stating "informed refusal for police intimation" should be made.
- Only in situations, where it is life-threatening the doctor may initiate treatment without consent as per Section 92 of IPC.
- The consent form must be signed by the person himself/herself if he/she is above 12 years of age.
- Consent must be taken from the guardian/parent if the survivor is under the age of 12 years.
- The consent form must be signed by the survivor, a witness and the examining doctor.

Two marks of identification such as moles, scars, tattoos, etc. preferably from the exposed parts of the body should be documented. While describing identification mark emphasis should be on size, site, surface, shape, colour, fixity to underlying structures. Left thumb impression is to be taken in the space provided.

ONE STOP CENTRE[2]

Introduction[2]

One stop centres (OSCs) are intended to support women affected by violence, in private and public spaces, within the family, community and at the workplace. Women facing physical, sexual, emotional, psychological and economic abuse, irrespective of age, class, caste, education status, marital status, race and culture will be facilitated with support and redressal.

Objectives[2]

1. To provide integrated support and assistance to women affected by violence, both in private and public spaces under one roof.
2. To facilitate immediate, emergency and non-emergency access to a range of services including medical, legal, psychological and counselling support under one roof to fight against any forms of violence against women.

Target Group[2]

- All women including girls below 18 years of age affected by violence, irrespective of caste, class, religion, region, sexual orientation or marital status.
- For girls below 18 years of age, institutions and authorities established under Juvenile Justice (Care and Protection of Children) Act, 2000 and the Protection of Children from Sexual Offences Act, 2012 will be linked with the OSC.

Location[2]

For establishing a centre

- The first preference would be to consider proposals where suitable and adequate accommodation with separate access having at least 5 rooms and carpet area of 132 sq.m. within a hospital/medical facility, that is prominently visible and easily accessible to the women affected by violence is available.
- If it is not possible, then an existing government/semi-government institutions/women institutions/Swadhar Grehs/working women hostels located within 2 km radius of the hospital/medical facility.

- If it is not feasible to locate the centre in the existing accommodation, the centres may be constructed on suitable land having at least an area of 300 sq.m. as identified by the state government.

Services[2]

The OSC will facilitate access to following services:
1. Emergency response and rescue services
2. Medical assistance
3. Assistance to women in lodging FIR/NCR/DIR
4. Psychosocial support/counselling
5. Legal aid and counselling
6. Shelter
7. Video conferencing facility

Service Delivery Framework: Roles and Responsibilities[2]

The service providers of the OSC will have following responsibilities.

Centre Administrator—the First Point of Contact

The centre administrator would be a woman with requisite qualification, a residential staff attached to OSC, would be in-charge of functioning of OSC.

Case Worker

She will provide assistance and support to the centre administrator in facilitating services to women accessing OSC.

Police Facilitation Officer (PFO)

a. Will help the aggrieved women in initiating appropriate police proceedings against the perpetrators and would help expedite the process and in special cases, flag the issue to the superintendent of police.
b. In case the aggrieved woman is unable to go to the police station for lodging her complaint/FIR, the police facilitation officer will ensure the recording of information from her home/OSC/hospital after obtaining due permissions.

Paralegal Personnel/Lawyer

Help/guide the woman to initiate legal proceedings against the abuse/violence suffered, if she is willing to do so and facilitate speedy and hassle free police and court proceedings.

Paramedical Personnel

First aid and immediate life-saving medical assistance to the aggrieved woman and accompany the woman.

Counsellor

Will provide psychological counselling.

IT Staff

Would generate the unique ID of the women affected, document the case history as provided, help in video conferencing, data entry operations, etc.

Multipurpose Helper

Would be responsible for maintaining hygiene and sanitation at OSC.

Security Guard/Night Guard

The security guard/night guard would be responsible for the overall security of OSC.

Diagrammatic Overview of One Stop Centre: Human Resource and Services.[2]

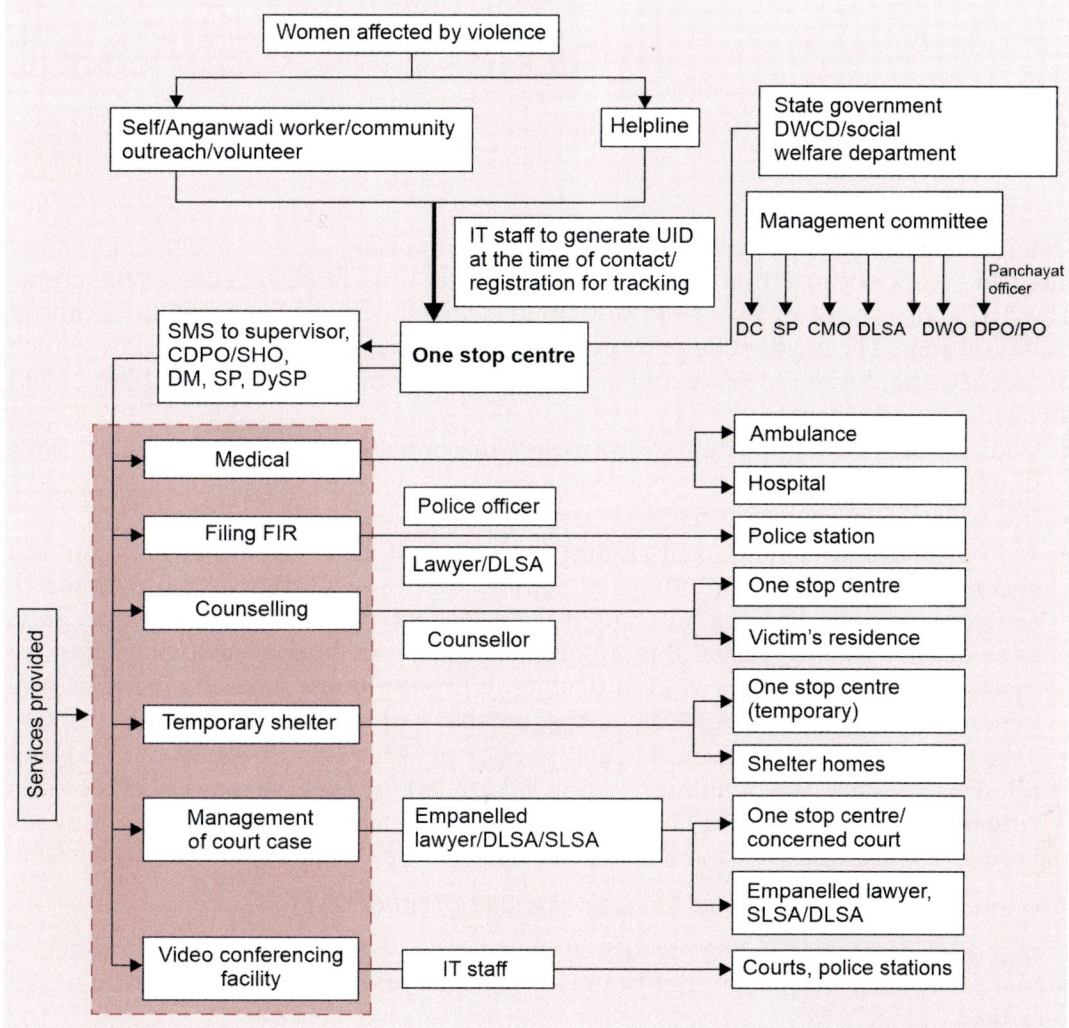

SLSA—State Legal Service Authority; DLSA—District Legal Service Authority; DC—District Commissioner; SP—Suprintendent of Police; CMO—Chief Medical Officer; DPO—District Programme Officer; PO—Protection Officer.

REFERENCES

1. MOHFW 2014 Guidelines and Protocols Medico-legal care for survivors/victims of sexual violence.
2. https://wcd.nic.in/schemes/one-stop-centre-scheme-1.

Determining the Age of Injuries in Sexual Assault

Meenakshi Deshpande

Determining the age of injuries is one of the most important aspects in clinical forensic medicine work because this aspect is related to the time of occurrence of the crime. The 2012 gang rape of a 23-year-old student in Delhi who died from her injuries caused public outrage. The incident helped spur an amendment to India's criminal law, which broadened the definition of sexual crimes against women to include stalking, acid attacks and voyeurism.

- Without accurate documentation and expert interpretation of injuries, any conclusions drawn can be flawed.
- It is of vital importance in the reconstruction of the chain of events.
- ACOG guidelines say: Sexual assault is a crime of violence and aggression and encompasses a continuum of sexual activity that ranges from sexual coercion to contact abuse and violence (unwanted kissing, touching, or fondling) to rape. *Rape*, as re-defined by the Federal Bureau of Investigation in 2013, is the penetration, no matter how slight, of the vagina or anus with any body part or object, or oral penetration or by a sex organ of another person, without the consent of the victim.
- This definition notably excludes any gender of victim and perpetrator and any reference to force. The definition acknowledges that rape and sexual assault occur in situations in which consent is not given, such as situations of intoxication or when individuals are otherwise mentally or physically incapable of demonstrating consent.

Are Injuries seen in Cases of Sexual Assault? (Figure 18.1)

Nongenital or genital **injury** occurs in about 50% of rapes of females. However, actual prevalence may be higher because rape and **sexual assault** tend to be under reported.[4]

- Although presence of injuries is not mandatory to prove sexual violence, 5% have moderate and 1% severe physical injury (head injuries, strangulation, fractures, widespread soft tissue injuries).
- The likelihood of significant genital injury is uncommon (except in pre-pubertal girls and post-menopausal women).
- Any suspicious injuries/wounds must be thought of as due to sexual abuse.
- Although many vulvar lacerations are the result of sports-related straddle-type injuries, genital trauma is reported in 20–53% of sexual assault victims.

- **Location and frequency of injury**

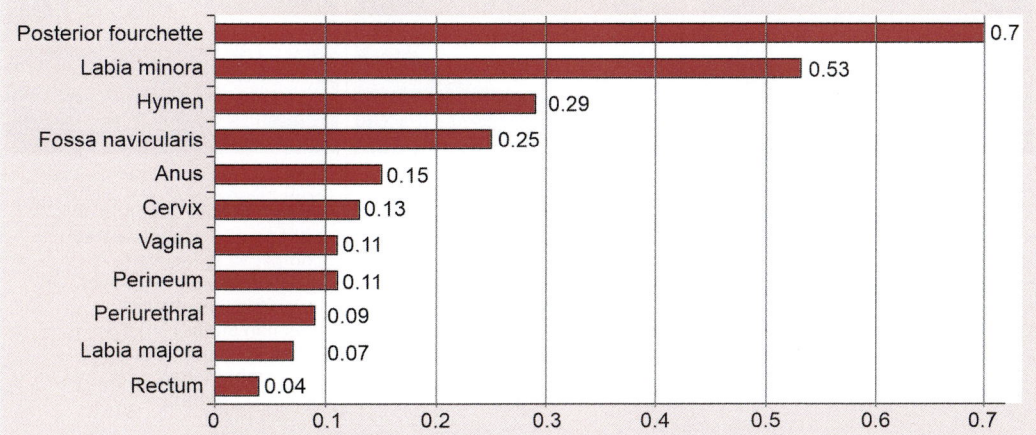

Figure 18.1: Sexual assault and general body injuries [a detailed cross-sectional Australian study of 1163 women]. (*Courtesy*: Forensic Science International Oct. 2017. Renate R Zilkens[a], Debbie A Smith[b], Maire C Kelly[b], S Aqif Mukhtar[a], James B Semmens[a], Maureen A Phillips[ab])

- Highlights: Detailed analysis shows the associations of body injury in female **sexual assault**
  - 1 in 5 women have moderate or severe injury after sexual assault.
  - Intimate partner sexual assaults have the greatest risk of any body injury.
  - Intimate partner sexual assaults also have the most risk of more severe body injury.

  Associations between body injury and assailant type varied by mental health status.

Evaluation and Assessment of Injuries

- Informed consent for the patient assessment should be obtained if a history of sexual assault has been verified. This consent format should include assessment by **detailed history, physical examination, and collection of laboratory and forensic specimens and photography** especially of injuries, wherever required as outlined by the American College of Obstetrics and Gynecologists.
- Doctors need to assess: The age of an injury; how (i.e. the mechanism by which) the injury was produced; the amount of force required to produce the injury; the circumstances in which the injury was sustained; the consequences of the injury so as to form a MLC report.
- Interpretation of injury requires expertise and is entirely dependent on the accuracy and completeness of the recorded observations of wounds (Figure 18.2).
- Health workers are advised to document and refer to forensic expert for interpretation to know the interpretation.
- MLC report is expected to narrate incident, details of injuries, time lapses. Interpretation by the doctor must correlate between said and actual findings, i.e. nature of violence, timings of injuries, why there was loss of evidence, any evidence of use of drugs/alcohol intoxication.
- Rape and sexual assault are legal terms. Doctors should not use them. When feasible, photographs of possible injuries are taken.

Inflammatory phase	Proliferative phase	Maturation phase
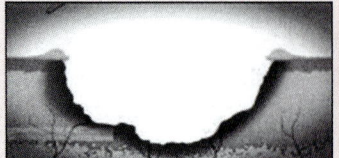	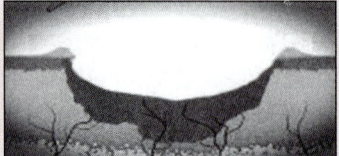	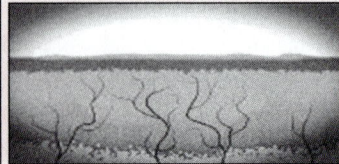
• Begins when the wound develops, last 4–6 days • Marked by oedema, erythema, inflammation and pain • Healing process triggered • Immune system works to prevent microbial colonization	• Lasts another 4–24 days • Granulation tissue fills in the wound • Fibroblasts lay collagen in the wound bed, strengthening new granulation tissue • Wound edges begin to contract • Epithelial cells migrate from the wound margins	• Can last 21 days to 2 years • Length of time depends on patient- and wound-related complicating factors (e.g. duration of wound, patient comorbidities, wound infection status) • Filled-in wound is covered and strengthened • Scar tissue forms

Figure 18.2: Phases of genital injury

- The following details about the alleged assault must be documented, preferably in an examination proforma:
  - the date, time and location of the assault, including
    - description of the type of surface on which the assault occurred;
    - the name, identity and number of assailants;
    - the nature of the physical contacts and detailed account of violence inflicted;
    - use of weapons and restraints;
    - use of medications/drugs/alcohol/inhaled substances; and
    - how clothing was removed.

The Physical Examination of Injuries

- Sequence is important
- Use universal precautions
- Warm, clean well lighted room with screen/adequate privacy
- If bleeding injuries—control bleeding by gauze
- Firstly check vital signs, i.e. blood pressure; temperature; pulse; respiration rate
- Patient's general appearance, demeanor and mental functioning
- Explain the procedure and instruments
- Chaperone/attendant/female relative must be present
- Examine the patient from head-to-toe, concluding with the genito-anal area (Figure 18.3)
- The pattern of injuries sustained during an incident of sexual violence may show considerable variation. This may range from complete absence of injuries (more frequently) to grievous injuries (very rare).
- Note and describe in detail any physical injuries, even if forensic evidence is not being collected.
- Use body maps to indicate location and size of injury
- Photograph any injuries. A separate consent form for photography may be necessary.

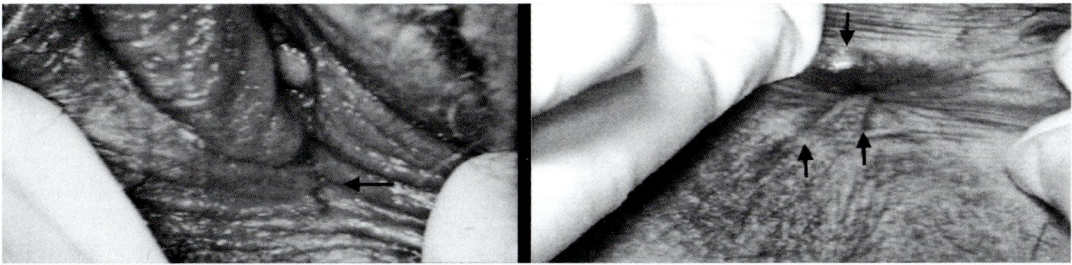

Figure 18.3: Genital anal injuries

- Please do not mention old scars as they are identification marks rather than new injuries due to assault. If mentioning those seems pertinent, add a note on when they were acquired.
- The mouth, breasts, genitals, and rectum are examined closely. Common sites of injury include the labia minora and posterior vagina.
- Examination using a Wood's lamp may detect semen or foreign debris on the skin.
- Colposcopy is particularly sensitive for subtle genital injuries. Some colposcopes have cameras attached, making it possible to detect and photograph injuries simultaneously. Whether use of toluidine blue to highlight areas of injury is accepted as evidence varies by jurisdiction.

Skin Wound Healing (Figure 18.4)

Skin wound healing is a primitive but well orchestrated biological phenomena consisting of three sequential phases, inflammation, proliferation, and maturation.

Many biological substances are involved in the process of wound repair, and this short and simplified overview of wound healing can be adopted to determine wound vitality or wound age in forensic medicine.

Inflammatory phase	Proliferative phase	Maturation phase
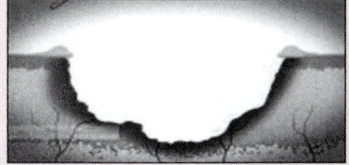	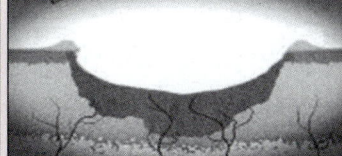	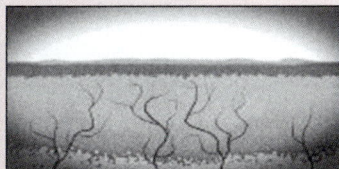
• Begins when the wound develops, last 4–6 days • Marked by oedema, erythema, inflammation and pain • Healing process triggered • Immune system works to prevent microbial colonization	• Lasts another 4–24 days • Granulation tissue fills in the wound • Fibroblasts lay collagen in the wound bed, strengthening new granulation tissue • Wound edges begin to contract • Epithelial cells migrate from the wound margins	• Can last 21 days to 2 years • Length of time depends on patient- and wound-related complicating factors (e.g. duration of wound, patient comorbidities, wound infection status) • Filled-in wound is covered and strengthened • Scar tissue forms

Figure 18.4: Phases of wound healing

Body Map for Charting (Figure 18.5)

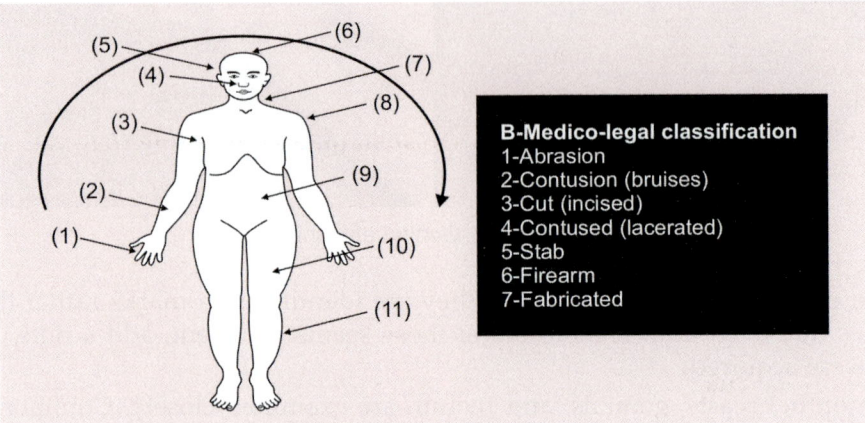

B-Medico-legal classification
1-Abrasion
2-Contusion (bruises)
3-Cut (incised)
4-Contused (lacerated)
5-Stab
6-Firearm
7-Fabricated

Figure 18.5: Body mapping

Types of Injuries and their Age Estimation

1. **Bruise/contusion** (Figure 18.6): Leakage or extravasation of blood from blood vessels in the skin and subcutaneous tissues, which have been disrupted by blunt force.
   - They can be petechial. These often arise from disruption of small venules, e.g. above site of strangulation, suction type injury
   - Trainline—struck with a rod-like object
   - Fingerpad—patterned

   These associated with:
   - Redness—could be from infection, inflammation or trauma
   - Tenderness—subjective

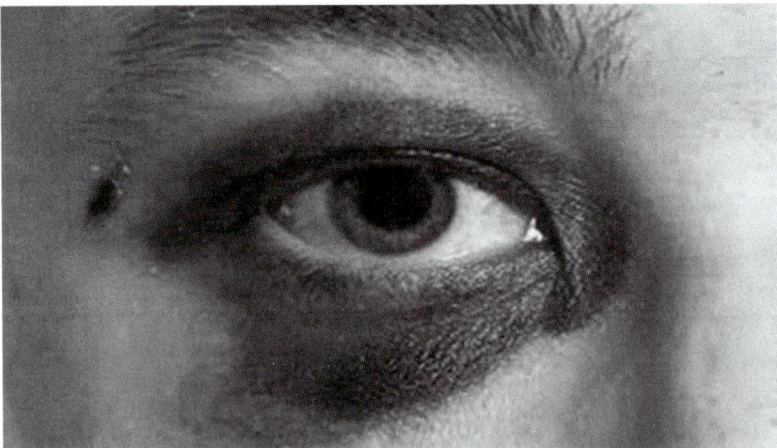

Figure 18.6: Bruises

Factors affecting development and appearance of a bruise
- Force of impact
- Duration of impact

- Site properties of body region impacted (blood supply, underlying bone, tissue planes)
- Quantity of blood extravasated
- Depth of bruise
- Age and health of individual (medications, coagulation status)
- Skin colour
    - **So, multiple bruises** (Figure 18.7) **sustained at the same time can all appear different**
    - The woman is examined again in one or two days later when new bruising may be more easily seen, and a comparison of the age of different bruises can be made.

Age of bruises: One cannot determine the age of a bruise. It is very subjective. Superficial bruises appear almost at once

- Deep bruises may not appear for hours/days
- Red may actually appear at any time
- Bruises of same age on same person may be different colours and may change at different rates.
- **The presence of yellow discoloration in a bruise indicates it is older than 18 hours**. No yellow does not mean bruise is less than 18 hours.

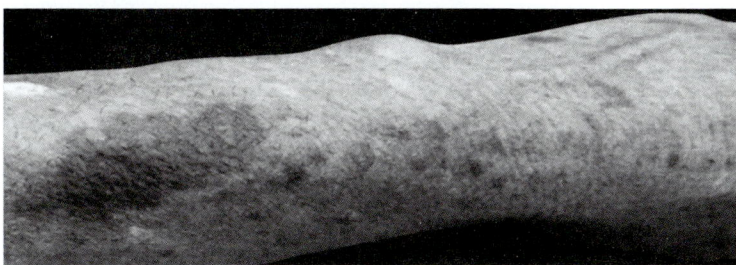

Figure 18.7: Multiple bruises

The age of bruise (Figure 18.8): The colour of the bruise may change with the age of the injury.

At first: The bruise appears bright red, tenderness and redness is present.

At few hours to 3 days: Blue discolouration.

On the 4th day: Bluish-black to brown discoloration due to haemosiderin pigment.

On the 5th to 6th days: Greenish discoloration due to haematoidin pigment.

On the 7th to 12th days: Yellow discoloration due to bilirubin.

At 2 weeks: Normal

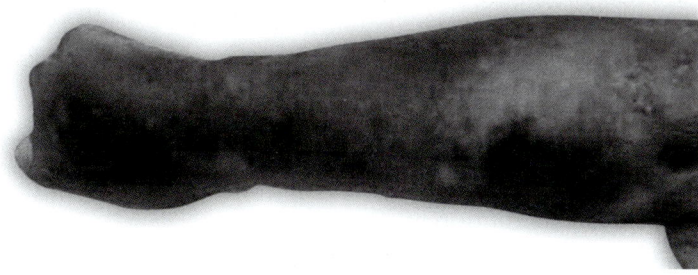

Figure 18.8: Bruises

2. **An abrasion:** It involves destruction of the skin, which usually involves the superficial layers of the epidermis only. They are caused by a lateral rubbing action by a blow, a fall on a rough surface, by being dragged in a vehicular accident, fingernails, thorns or teeth bite.
   - Abrasions are of four types:
     1. Scratches; 2. Grazes; 3. Pressure abrasions; 4. Impact abrasions

   Age of the abrasions (Figure 18.9)**: The exact age cannot be determined**
   - Fresh abrasions: Bright red, painful, oozing.
   - At 12 to 24 hours: It appears bright red to dark red. A reddish scab appears. lymph and blood dries up leaving a bright scab.
   - At 2 to 3 days: Reddish-brown scab.
   - At 7 days: Epithelium grows and covers defect under the scab. Then it starts falling
   - After 7 days: Scab dries, shrinks and falls off leaving depigmented area underneath.

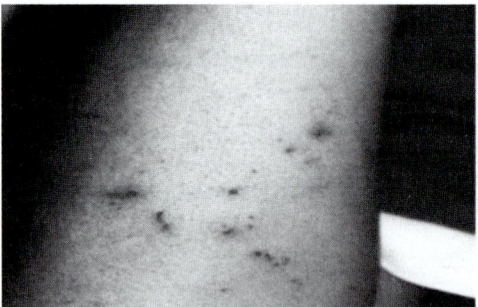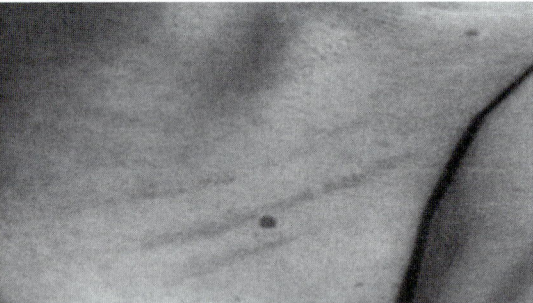

Figure 18.9: Abrasions

3. **Incised wounds:** Incised wound is clean cut through the tissues caused with sharp edged weapon, which is longer than its depth. Produced when any sharp edged weapon, e.g. knife, end of a metal sheet, piece of a broken glass drawn across the skin.
   1. Margins: Length is the greatest dimension
      - Margins are clean cut, well defined and there is no bruising
      - All tissues are evenly divided
      - Blood vessels cleanly cut: No tissue bridges
   2. Width: Width greater than edge of the weapon
   3. Length: Length or depth has no relation to cutting edge
   4. Shape: Spindle-shaped or zigzag (if skin is lax) or crescentic (curved blade)
   5. Hemorrhage is more (vessel cut), spurting in arterial bleeding
   6. Direction: Deeper at beginning (head) and shallow at end (tailing)

   Age of incised wound
   - Fresh—hematoma formation
   - 12 hours—edges swollen, red, adherent with blood and lymph, leucocytic infiltration
   - 24 hours—continuous epithelial layer covers the surface of clot

Histopathology of age changes with time since injury as follows:

- Few minutes: Capillaries dilation, margination and migration of neutrophils, swelling of endothelium.
- 12 hours: Reactive changes in fibroblasts, monocytes appear
- 24 hours: Epithelium begins to grow at edges
- 72 hours: Vascularized granulation tissue
- 4–5 days: New fibrils formed
- 7 days: Scar formation

4. **Laceration:** Result from the application of a blunt force which causes splitting or tearing of the skin and/or subcutaneous tissues.

Age of lacerated/stab wound

- Unsutured: Inflammed edges—up to 24 hours. Appearance of infection—more than 36 hours.
- Sutured:
  - Inflammed edges—up to 24 hours
  - Edges easily separated—1–3 days
  - Edges difficult to separate—3–7 days
  - Red soft tender scar—1 to 4 weeks
  - Pale firm nontender scar—more than 4 weeks

5. **Chopped wounds:** Chop wounds are deep gaping wounds caused with sharp splitting edge of heavy weapons like axe, sword, meat cleaver, etc.

Appearance of chopped wounds have the following features

- Dimension depends on the cross-section of weapon
- Margins moderately sharp
- They are usually with abrasions and bruises
- There may be destruction of underlying tissue and organs
- Depth may be same throughout
- Mostly seen on head, face, neck, shoulders and extremities
- There may be injuries to underlying bones
- Majority are homicidal, few accidental recovered from water propellers of boats
- Rarely suicidal
- Microscopy helps to determine antemortem nature.

SOURCE REFERENCES AND SUGGESTED READING

1. Assessment and examination of adult victims of sexual violence https://www.who.int › resources › publications › guidelines_chap 4.
2. Examination for sexual assault: Is the documentation of physical injury associated with the laying of charges? A retrospective cohort study Margaret J. McGregor, MD, MHSc; Grace Le, MD, MHSc; Stephen A. Marion, MD, MHSc; Ellen Wiebe, MD.
3. Forensic sexual assault examination and genital injury: is skin...Https://www.ncbi.nlm.nih.gov › pmc › articles › pmc2587067Bymssommers-?2008.
4. MSD _ Manuals/revision October 2017 by Erin G. Clifton, PhD.
5. A review and study of the colour changes with time [For Sci.Int 1991].
6. Examination of A Injured Person.pdfwww.kimsmedicalcollege.org.

Management and Treatment of Domestic Violence

Meka Krishna Kumari

'**Domestic violence**' is violence or abuse happening when it is associated with a close relationship between the offender and the victim and includes partners and ex-partners, immediate family members, other relatives and family friends.

It includes any injuries which affect a woman's mental, sexual, reproductive and physical health, safety, or her well-being.

According to United Nation Population Fund, in India, four in ten married women and nearly 35% of women between the ages of 15 and 49 suffer from some form of domestic violence. It is under-reported with less than 40% of women who have experienced violence seeking help. Over 30% women suffered physical and sexual violence by their spouses in five out of 22 surveyed states and Union Territories according to the National Family Health Survey 5 (2019-2020) with several outliers and rural/urban divide.[1]

The prevalence that has been reported during pregnancy is approximately 30% emotional abuse, 15% physical abuse, and 8% sexual abuse on an average. Domestic violence occurs in gay, lesbian, bisexual, and transgender couples, and the rates are thought to be similar to a heterosexual woman, approximately 25%. The methods used are either coercion, threats, intimidation, isolating or emotionally abusing them, controlling the woman by using finances, children or male aggressiveness.

Women more at risk are:

- Young age, illiteracy, financial dependence
- Infertility/bearing female children
- Pregnancy—with abdomen usually being targeted
- Chronic ill health and disability
- Previous history of domestic violence or sexual assault
- Substance abuse/mental ill health of the perpetrator

The survivors of sexual violence may present to either the emergency room, or to the outpatient department. The three basic components of health response include collecting evidence, clinical care and appropriate referral. They may present to health care services with varying signs and symptoms and often have unnecessary investigations and medication for nonspecific or mental health symptoms.

The examining physician has to proactively be on the lookout for symptoms and signs of domestic violence for these survivors who do not reveal a history of sexual violence.

Obstetrician and gynecologists are in a unique position to assess and provide support for women who experience intimate partner violence (IPV) because of the nature of the patient–physician relationship and the many opportunities for intervention that come during the course of pregnancy, family planning, annual examinations, and other women's health visits.[2]

The following signs and symptoms should prompt one to suspect the possibility of sexual abuse/assault:

Physical markers

- Severe abdominal/pelvic pain.
- Sexual dysfunction/dyspareunia.
- Menstrual disorders.
- Burning micturition/urinary tract infections.
- Chronic gastrointestinal symptoms.
- Chronic headache.
- Unwanted pregnancy/miscarriage/unsafe abortion/high risk pregnancies/ increased maternal morbidity and mortality.
- Exposure to sexually transmitted infections (including HIV/AIDS).
- Somatic symptom disorder
- Pelvic inflammatory disease
- Infertility
- Genital mutilation
- Repeated consultations.

Psychological markers

- Fear and shock.
- Physical and emotional pain or numbing.
- Intense self-disgust/denial.
- Feeling of worthlessness and powerlessness.
- Generalised apathy and withdrawal.
- An inability to function normally in their daily lives.
- Depression and chronic anxiety.
- Self-blame/feelings of vulnerability.
- Loss of control/loss of self-esteem.
- Emotional distress.
- Nightmares.
- Mistrust.
- Avoidance
- Post-traumatic stress disorder and chronic mental disorders.
- Committing suicide or endangering their lives.

Health care professionals have a responsibility ethically to recognize and manage exposure to abuse in their patients.

"Due to the prevalence and medical consequences of family violence, physicians should routinely inquire about physical, sexual, and psychological abuse as part of the medical history.

Physicians must also consider abuse in the differential diagnosis for a number of medical complaints, particularly when treating women as per the "American Medical Association's code of medical ethics."

The acronym **LIVES** has been used by WHO for guiding health care providers as first line response to support women who suffered domestic violence:[3] **L**: Listen closely, with empathy and no judgement; **I**: Inquire about their needs and concerns; **V**: Validate their experiences; **E**: Enhance their safety; **S**: Support them to connect with additional services.

Management

- Treatment of survivors
- Preventing repetitions of such violence.

Treatment

Physical/sexual injuries. Emotional/psychological injuries

It is not mandatory for a survivor/victim of sexual violence to go to a government hospital for medical examination.

Section 357C of CrPC mandates all hospitals, irrespective of whether they are government, public sector or private sector, to immediately provide first aid and medical treatment free of cost.

Primarily note if she has been previously examined elsewhere. If so, if the survivor is carrying any documentation. The information has to be kept confidential. Individual's privacy has to be respected. Prior consent has to be taken.

Treatment Components

- Provide first aid and treat physical injuries
- STI prevention/treatment
- Vaccinations: Tetanus, hepatitis B
- Post-exposure prophylaxis
- Emergency contraception/safe abortion where necessary
- Counselling
- Any other

Management of the Survivor (Figure 19.1)

- The priority is the ABCs and appropriate treatment of the presenting complaints. After the patient is stabilized, emergency medical services personnel may identify other violence associated problems.
- Safe environment for the survivor has to be provided.
- Look for physical injuries and associated medical or surgical problems.
- The sources of domestic violence have to be identified.
- Is domestic violence the diagnosis?
- Reassuring the patient and evaluating the emotional status followed by treatment.

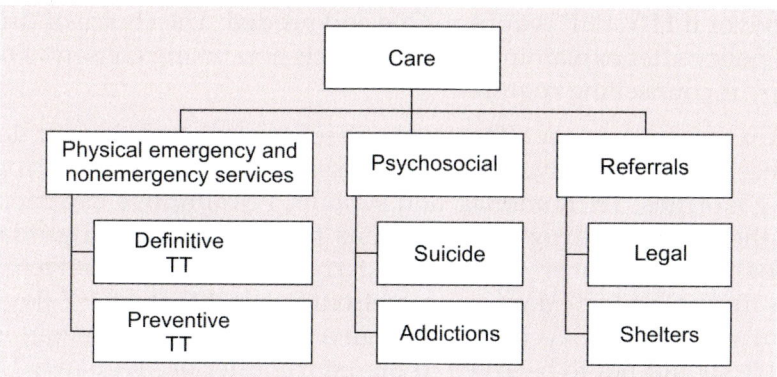

Figure 19.1: Algorithm for management

- Documentation of the history, physical examination, and interventions.
- Assess the risks to the victim and possible safety options.
- Counsel the patient regarding future violence.
- Determine if legal intervention is needed and report abuse when appropriate or mandated.
- A follow-up plan has to be developed.
- Offer shelter options, legal services, counseling, and facilitate referrals if required.

Injuries in domestic violence are usually central and need to be immediately treated or referred to a specialist. The most commonest sites of injury are areas usually covered by clothing (e.g. chest, breast, abdomen) and the face, neck, throat and genitalia. Maxillofacial trauma includes injuries to the eye and ear, soft tissues, hearing loss, loss of vision, and fractures of the mandible, nasal bones, orbits, and zygomaticomaxillary complex.

Lacerations: Clean with antiseptic or soap and water. If there are injuries and survivor is not immunized, administer ½ cc TT IM. If lacerations require repair and suturing, surgical treatment is to be done.

Emergency contraception: Emergency contraception has to be offered to survivors of sexual assault presenting within 5 days of sexual assault, ideally as soon as possible after the assault for maximum effectiveness. A single dose of 1.5 mg levonorgestrel is recommended, or two doses of 0.75 mg given 12–24 hours apart. If vomiting occurs, repeat within 3 hours. OR COCs are to be used, a split dose, one dose of 100 µg of ethinyl estradiol plus 0.50 mg of LNG, followed by a second dose 12 hours later (Yuzpe method) with antiemetics to minimise nausea and vomiting may be given. If ongoing contraception is needed, IUCD insertion can be done within 5 days of the assault as per the medical eligibility criteria. Pregnancy assessment must be done on follow-up and the survivor must be advised to get tested for pregnancy in case she misses her next period.

Safe abortion: If a woman presents after the time required for emergency contraception (5 days) or emergency contraception fails, or the woman is pregnant as a result of rape, pregnancy test is to be done and she should be offered safe abortion, in accordance with national MTP law.

HIV post-exposure prophylaxis (PEP): Consider offering HIV post-exposure prophylaxis for women presenting within 72 hours of a sexual assault. Use shared decision-making with the survivor if HIV PEP is appropriate and needed. The choice of drugs is as per the national policy after explaining the side-effects and taking consent. For adherence to the therapy is counselling required.

Post-exposure prophylaxis for STIs: In the presence of clinical signs or depending on the prevalence, women survivors of sexual assault may be offered prophylaxis for Chlamydia, gonorrhea, Trichomonas, and syphilis. Presumptive treatment should be given with the choice of drug and regimens following national guidance for the organism. For non-pregnant women, the preferred choice is azithromycin 1 gm stat or doxycycline 100 mg bd for 7 days, with metronidazole 400 mg for 7 days with food. For pregnant women, amoxycillin/azithromycin with metronidazole is preferred. Metronidazole should not to be given in the 1st trimester of pregnancy.[4]

Hepatitis B vaccination without hepatitis B immunoglobulin should be offered as per national guidelines after checking for immune status.

Psychological effects include evaluation and treatment of the survivor's emotional status. They suffer with:

- Feeling of disassociation from her body or reality, or both
- Eidetic memory—photographic flashbacks and experiencing the memories
- Recall—retrieval of her previous memories completely
- Hyperarousal of the autonomic nervous system
- Hypervigilance—paranoid level of fear or mistrust, or intense awareness of every word and Act, and a distorted sense of time

Studies show that some form of individual cognitive behavioural therapy (CBT) interventions for women who have experienced intimate partner violence may reduce post-traumatic stress disorder and depression. Women with a pre-existing mental disorder or suffering from violence related mental disorder (such as depression, or alcohol use disorder) and are experiencing violence should receive mental health care including antidepressants under specialist care.

Women centered care: Women who disclose any form of violence by an intimate partner (or other family member) or sexual assault by any perpetrator should be offered immediate support and comprehensive services that focuss on her needs and requirements.

One stop centres: They are government sponsored centres for addressing the problem of violence against women which provide integrated support and assistance to women affected with violence under one roof. They provide a full range of services including police, prosecutors, social worker, counsellors, psychological support, etc.

Health care for women subjected to intimate partner violence or sexual violence. Geneva: World Health Organization; 2014 (http://www.who.int/reproductive health/publications/violence/VAW-clinical-handbook/en/).

The next step after primary care includes counselling and future planning: Counselling the individual, family and couple counselling. Counselling of the offender: Lethality assessment, safety planning, anger management, follow-up—next visit, rehabilitation—yoga and meditation, occupational therapy. Prevention—short stay homes or shelter homes may help.

Care of survivors is a continuum (Figure 19.2).

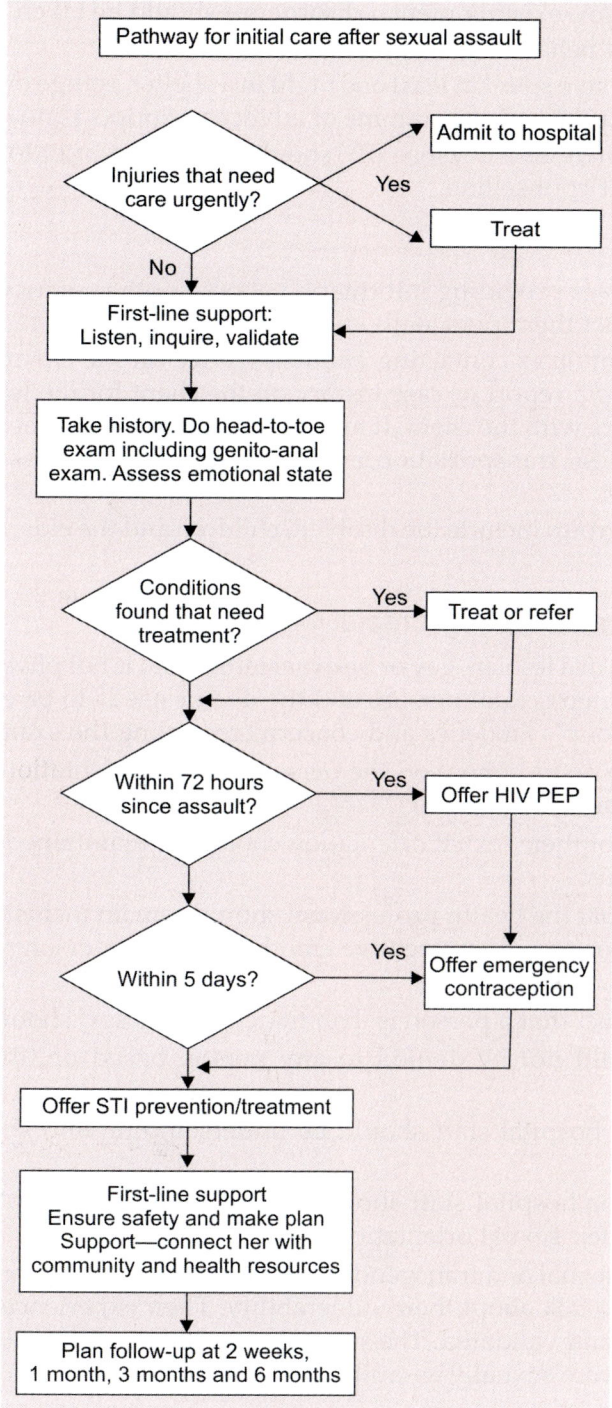

Figure 19.2: Further plan of treatment

Follow-up: Review for STIs if possible. Test for pregnancy.

• Assess for psychological sequelae and re-iterate need for psychological support as the risk of depression nearly doubles up.

- Women with pre-existing mental disorders—should be taken care appropriately
- Cognitive and behavior therapy
- Women who have spent at least one night in a shelter, refuge or safe house should be offered a structured programme of advocacy, support and/or empowerment.
- Pregnant women who disclose IPV should be offered brief to medium duration empowerment counselling.

Referral

Cold referral involves providing information about another agency or service so that the client can contact them personally.

Warm referral involves contacting another service on the client's behalf and may also involve writing a report or case history on the client for the legal service and/or attending the service with the client. It may be appropriate in women who lack reliable internet/phone access, transportation, and housing, and lack access to social, financial, and other supports.

The vulnerable group include the disabled, children and the elderly and need special attention.

Guidelines for Examination of Special Groups[5]

- The examination of a lesbian, gay or bisexual individual is not physically any different from that of a heterosexual person, and the doctor needs to be especially sensitive to the former group's anxieties and concerns regarding the examinations.
- There should be no judgment on the person's sexual orientation in general or as a cause of the assault.
- Confidentiality of their sexual orientation should be maintained unless needed for treatment reasons.
- It is important that the health professional should remain inclusive and not express shock, wonder, or any other negative emotions when a person reveals their sexual orientation.
- Old injuries or fact that a person is 'habituated to anal sex' should not be recorded.
- Treatment should not be denied to any person based on/due to their sexual orientation.
- The doctor and hospital staff should be understanding and should provide care and treatment.
- The doctor or the hospital staff should not give any advice or 'offer solutions' to 'cure' them of their sexual orientation.
- Lesbian, gay, bisexual and transgender persons are likely to be targets of hate crimes and may want to talk about their vulnerability. Their experience should be given a sincere hearing and validated. The survivors should be assured that it was not their fault that they were sexually assaulted.

Caring for children who witness DV: Approximately 10% of children are exposed to domestic violence annually, and 25% are exposed to at least 1 event during their childhood. These children are prone for increased risk of post-traumatic stress disorder, aggressive behavior, anxiety, impaired development, difficulty interacting with peers, academic problems, and they have a higher incidence of substance abuse.

Occupational therapy and financial independence play an important role. The most common problem areas were leisure, education, work, child rearing, and health management.[6] Economic independence is achieved by combining microfinance with developing decision-making skills regarding employment opportunities, skills training, stress management, time, money and home management, communication and interpersonal skills, improving self-esteem, active social participation and lifestyle modification to establish healthy routines.

Domestic violence in COVID times: Peace is not just the absence of war. Many women under lockdown for COVID-19 face violence where they should be the safest in their own homes.

—**UN Chief Antonio Gutteres**

Stress, the disruption of social and protective networks, women locked at home, loss of income and decreased access to services all can exacerbate the risk of violence for women. There has been a reduction in survivors seeking services due to a combination of lockdown measures and not wanting to attend health services for fear of infection.

To summarize the pathway to care includes:

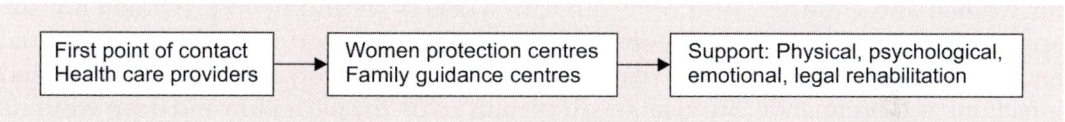

The only way to break the cycle of domestic violence is to break the silence, Act, ensure economic independence, and have a robust integrated national plan including health care personnel.

REFERENCES

1. World Health Organization. Fact sheets, Key facts. 2019; Available from: https://www.who.int/en/news-room/fact-sheets/detail/malaria.
2. Committee on Obstetric Practice. Committee opinion. Obstet Gynecol. 2002;99(4):679–80.
3. WHO. Responding to intimate partner violence and sexual violence against women. 2011; Available from: www.who.int/reproductivehealth.
4. Redfield RR, Bunnell R, Ellis B, Kent CK, Leahy MA, Martinroe JC, et al. Recommendations for Providing Quality Sexually Transmitted Diseases Clinical Services, 2020. Centers for Disease Control and Prevention. Centers Dis Control Prev. 2020;68(5).
5. Violence S. Guidelines & protocols, medical examination and reporting for sexual violence arogya. maharashtra.gov.in.
6. Javaherian-Dysinger H, Krpalek D, Huecker E, Hewitt L, Cabrera M, Brown C, Francis J, Rogers K, Server S. Occupational Needs and Goals of Survivors of Domestic Violence. Occup Ther Health Care. 2016;30(2):175-86. doi: 10.3109/07380577.2015.1109741. Epub 2015 Dec 8. PMID: 26647100.

Medical and Surgical Management in Sexual Assault Case

Shilpa N Naik

Abstract

Sexual violence is a significant cause of physical and psychosocial harm and suffering for women and children. Aim of health care workers should be to provide a holistic approach and create a favourable environment for examination and treatment of sexual and domestic violence victims. Treatment includes prevention of sexually transmitted infections and pregnancy. Surgical repair of injuries on the perineum and deep wounds must be undertaken only after collection of important evidence. Counselling and psychological support is one of the mainstay of management of victims.

Management of victims of sexual assault are discussed under following heads:
- General management of victims of sexual assault
- Evaluation and management of survivors of sexual assault
- Pregnancy prevention and management, emergency contraception
- Infectious disease prevention and prophylaxis for STI and treatment
- Post-exposure prophylaxis for HIV
- Hepatitis B vaccination
- Psychological consequences
- Surgical management and postoperative care
- Patient follow-up
- Counseling
- Referrals

Evaluation and Management of Survivors of Sexual Assault

- Thorough gynecological examination is done after written informed consent from the victim herself in a case of major and from concerned guardian in a case of a minor.
- Assessment and treatment of injuries along with the forensic expert
- Obtain appropriate specimens and serology tests for STI testing before disinfecting and cleaning injury sites to avoid loss of evidence. This is the most important step.
- Provide appropriate prophylaxis for infectious disease like HIV, HbsAg and other sexually transmitted infections by following methods.

The following medications may be indicated:
- Antibiotics to prevent wounds from becoming infected;
- A tetanus booster or vaccination (according to local protocols);

- Medications for the relief of pain, anxiety or insomnia.
- Provide or arrange for provision of pregnancy prevention by providing emergency contraception
- Counsel about findings, recommendations and prognosis
- Arrange for follow-up medical care and referrals for psychological needs.

Pregnancy Prevention and Management

Female victims of sexual assault are concerned about pregnancy.

Hence, emergency contraceptives are offered if she presents within 5 days and if she presents more than 5 days after the assault she should be advised to return for pregnancy testing if she misses her next menstrual period.[1]

Following are the emergency contraceptive regimens used:

Up to 95% pregnancies can be prevented if used within 5 days.

Levonorgestrel 1.5 mg single dose.

Combined oral contraceptives (Yuzpe method)

100 µg ethinyl estradiol + 0.5 mg levonorgestrel 2 doses 12 hours apart.

Centchroman/ormeloxifen 2 tablets 50 mg 12 hours apart within 72 hours

Mifepristone: Single dose of 10 mg

Intrauterine device: Inserted up to 5 days of assault if desires on going contraception

Ulipristal acetate 30 mg single dose.

Instructions given to Victim Consuming ECP

ECPs are not 100% effective, possibility of pregnancy is there and minor side effects like nausea, vomiting and breast tenderness, spotting or bleeding could be there, but symptoms are mild and usually are brief in duration.

Pregnancy Testing and Management

- Pregnancy kits and ultrasound facilities are available for confirmation. If pregnancy is confirmed, victim is counselled regarding the same and informed about rights and options of termination or continuation of pregnancy.
- Choices about emergency contraception and pregnancy termination are personal and can be made by patient herself.
- Sexually transmitted infections

Common are Chlamydia, gonorrhoea, syphillis, trichomoniasis. Also look for HPV, HSV-2, HIV, hepatitis B.

WHO recommended STI treatment regimens (may also be used for prophylaxis).

Gonorrhoea	Cetriaxone or Cefixime	125 mg IM single dose 400 mg oral single dose
Chlamydia	Erythromycin Amoxicillin Azithromycin	500 mg QDS × 7 days 500 mg TDS × 7 days 1 g oral single dose
Syphilis	Benzathine penicillin or erythromycin	2.4 million in single dose 500 mg QDS × 14 days
Trichomonas and bactrial vaginosis	Metronidazole	2 g orally as a single dose or 1 g every 12 hours × 1 day

HIV Testing and Post-exposure Prophylaxis

Victims should be offered baseline HIV tests and counseled regarding confidentiality of tests.

Post-exposure prophylaxis should be initiated within 72 hours and is given for 28 days. Patient needs to be informed about:
- The limited data regarding the efficacy of PEP
- Possible side effects of the medications
- The need for strict compliance when taking the medications
- Length of treatment
- Importance of follow-up
- The need to begin treatment immediately.

Hepatitis B Transmission and Prevention

Victims are at risk of hepatitis B. Thus, testing should be offered when victim's vaccination status is not known.

Hepatitis B immunoglobulin 0.06 ml/kg is used anytime up to 72 hours after sexual Act when perpetrator is known to have active disease.[4]

When perpetrator is known to be hepatitis B positive and victim is known to be unvaccinated HIBG and vaccines are administered simultaneously at separate sites.

Patient Immunization Status and Treatment Guidelines

Never vaccinated for hepatitis B : 3 doses given at 0, 1 and 6 months
Not completed vaccination : Complete the scheduled
Completed a series of vaccination : No need to re-vaccinate

Psychological Effects and Consequences[5]

Psychological effects vary from person to person and commonly seen include:
- Rape trauma syndrome
- Post-traumatic stress disorder
- Depression
- Social phobias (especially in marital or date rape victims)
- Anxiety
- Increased substance use or abuse
- Suicidal behavior

In the long-term, victims may complain of the following:
- Chronic headaches
- Fatigue
- Sleep disturbances (i.e. nightmares, flashbacks)
- Sexual difficulties.

Rape Trauma Syndrome

Defined as "the stress response pattern of a person who has experienced sexual violence."

RTS may be manifested in somatic, cognitive, psychological and/or behavioral symptoms and usually consists of two phases: The acute phase and the long-term phase.[9]

Acute Phase

- The acute phase is a period of disorganization.
- Begins immediately and persists for 2–3 weeks.
- During the acute phase, a person usually experiences strong emotional reactions and may present with physical symptoms. Emotional responses include:
  - Crying and sobbing
  - Smiling and laughing
  - Calm and very controlled
  - A fat affect

The Long-term Phase

The subsequent phase is one of reorganization:

- Begins approximately 2–3 weeks after the event where.
- At this time the person starts to reorganize their lifestyle in adaptive or unadaptive way.
- This reorganization may be either adaptive or maladaptive
- Reactions during this phase vary markedly from person to person which include lifestyle changes difficulties in functioning at work, home or school and phobias, such as fear of crowds or a fear of being alone. Also sexual problems are noted.

Post-traumatic Stress Disorder (PTSD)

PTSD appears to be more common in persons who were threatened with a weapon and/or extreme physical force, in those raped by strangers, and in cases where physical injuries were inflicted.[8]

Symptoms of PTSD may manifest as intrusions involving flashback, nightmares, recurrent, intrusive thoughts that stay in the mind.

Avoidance symptoms include feelings of numbness, self-imposed isolation from family, friends and peers, increased drug or alcohol use, engaging in high-risk behaviors, avoiding places, activities or people that remind them of the assault.

Surgical Management of Injuries

- Obtain detailed history including gynecological history
- Obtain informed consent
- Perform physical examination including pelvic examination under good light setting
- Obtain appropriate specimens and serology tests for STI testing before disinfecting and cleaning injury sites (to avoid loss of evidence).
- Wounds are generally classified as either abrasion, bruises, lacerations, incisions, stab wounds or gunshot wounds.

  Describe wounds under following headings—size, site, shape, surroundings, colour, course, age, borders and depth.

Genito-anal Injuries Related to Penetration

- Trauma to the female genitalia and anus can be caused by forceful penetration.
- The posterior fourchette, the labia minora and majora, the hymen and the perianal folds are the most likely sites for injury, and abrasions, bruises.
- Lacerations are the most common forms of injury.

- Major injuries include rupture of perineal body, 3rd and 4th degree perineal tears, vulval haematoma, torn fornices, need for colostomy specially in child victims Genital injuries are recorded and classified under following headings:
    - The age of an injury
    - How (i.e. the mechanism by which) the injury was produced?
    - The amount of force required to produce the injury
    - The circumstances in which the injury was sustained
    - The consequences of the injury
    - Without accurate documentation and expert interpretation of injuries, any conclusions should not be drawn.

Steps of routine genito-anal examination

Step 1

- The external areas of the genital region and anus, thighs and buttocks should be examined for any markings.
- Inspect the mons pubis, vaginal vestibule paying special attention to the labia majora, labia minora, clitoris, hymen or hymenal remnants, fourchette and perineum.
- Swabs should be taken before any digital exploration or speculum examination.

Step 2

If any bright blood is present, it should be gently swabbed in order to establish its origin, i.e. whether it is vulval or from higher.

Step 3

- A speculum examination done to inspect the vaginal walls for signs of injury, foreign bodies and hair, may be found and collected. The endocervical canal can also be visualized. The duckbill speculum is used with patient in the lithotomy position which avoids any contact with the urethra, which is painful, and allows the cervix to be visualized with ease.
- In assaults that occurred more than 24 hours but less than 96 hours, prior to the physical examination, a speculum examination should be performed in order to collect an endocervical canal swab.

Step 4

Anal examination is performed in the patient in left lateral position. Respectful covering of the thighs and vulva with a gown or sheet during this procedure can help prevent a feeling of exposure. The uppermost buttock needs to be lifted to view the anus. Gentle pressure at the anal verge may reveal bruises, lacerations and abrasions.

Step 5

Digital rectal examinations are recommended if there is a suspect of foreign object inserted in the anal canal, and should be performed prior to a proctoscopy or anoscopy. Examination should be done after adequate relaxation of sphincters.

Step 6

Proctoscopy need only be used in cases of anal bleeding.[6]

Surgical Management Principles

- It is a multi-disciplinary approach
- Involve appropriate faculties like general surgeon, plastic surgeon, uro-surgeon, pediatrician, pediatric surgeon, forensic experts.

Mild to moderate injuries can be managed as follows:
- Antibiotics for preventing wound infection
- Tetanus vaccination or booster
- Pain management
- Surgical repair as per the injury
- Severe, life-threatening injuries: Refer to tertiary centre for management.

Surgical Care

- Thorough cleaning using pulse irrigations of 5% povidone iodine solution ± debridement
- Urethral catheterization using Foley catheter
- Approximation of torn vaginal muscles
- Vaginal mucosal suturing
- Trans anal repair of rectal mucosal injuries
- Sphincteric reconstruction and repair of the perineal body
- Labial reconstruction
- Diverting colostomy

Postoperative Care

- Intravenous antibiotics for 7–14 days
- Close follow-up for signs of wound infection: Charting of fever, hemogram, etc.
- Alternate day examinations after repair and pulse irrigations with antiseptic solution
- Warm seitz bath twice daily
- Colostomy care

Patient Information and Follow-up Care

- Give the patient ample opportunity to voice questions and concerns.
- Reassure the patient that the assault was not her fault.

Give patients written documentation regarding:
- Any treatments received or tests performed
- Date and time to call for test results
- Date and time of follow-up appointments
- Information regarding the legal process.

Follow-up care
- Medical review: Follow-up visits are recommended at 2 weeks for a duration of 3 months and 6 months post assault.
- 2-week follow-up visit

The following routine check up should be performed:
- Examine any injuries for proper healing
- Obtain cultures and draw blood to assess
- STI status
- Test for pregnancy if indicated. If pregnant, advise about options
- Remind patients for their hepatitis B vaccinations and HIV testing
- Encourage the patient to seek counseling 3-month and 6-month follow-up visits

- Test for HIV and make sure that pre- and post-testing counseling is available
- Draw blood for syphilis testing if prophylactic antibiotics were not given
- Encourage the patient to seek counselling if they have not yet done so.
- Administer the third dose of the hepatitis B vaccine at 6th month visit.

Counseling and Social Support

- Psychological counseling required varies depending on the degree of psychological trauma suffered and the victim's own coping skills and abilities
- The following approaches may be useful:
  - Listen carefully to the history of the event, ask about victim's concerns and address them appropriately
  - Reinforce that the assault was not victim's fault
  - Stress that sexual violence is an issue of power and control.
- Crisis intervention, critical incident stress debriefing, cognitive-behavioral therapy and feminist therapy are all forms of treatment that have been reported to work well with sexual assault victims.
- Save model protocol for survivors of sexual assault.

Patient should be given appropriate support services referrals which include rape crisis centers, shelters or safe houses, HIV/AIDS counselling, legal aid, victim witness programs, support groups, therapists, financial assistance agencies, social services agencies.

SOURCE REFERENCES AND SUGGESTED READING

1. Emergency contraceptive pills medical and service delivery guidelines. Seattle, WA, Consortium for Emergency Contraception, 2000.
2. Guidelines for the management of sexually transmitted infections. Geneva, World Health Organization (documents WHO/RHR/03.18, WHO/HIV/2003.09). In preparation.
3. Tjaden P, Thoennes N. Full report of the prevalence, incidence, and consequences of violence against women: findings from the National Violence Against Women Survey. Washington, DC, Office of Justice Programs, National Institute of Justice, 2000 (report number NCJ 183781. Bamberger JD, et al. Post-exposure prophylaxis for human immunodeficiency virus (HIV) infection following sexual assault. American Journal of Medicine, 1999, 106:323–26.
4. Doedens W. Clinical management of rape survivors: guide to assist in the development of situation-specific protocols. Geneva, World Health Organization, 2001 (document WHO/RHR/02.08).
5. Watts C, Zimmerman C. Violence against women: global scope and magnitude. Lancet, 2002, 359:1232–1237. Stevens L. A practical approach to gender-based violence: a programme guide for health care.
6. Welborn A. Adult sexual assault. Monash, Victoria, Monash University, 2000.
7. jaden P, Thoennes N. Full report of the prevalence, incidence, and consequences of violence against women: findings from the National Violence Against Women Survey. Washington, DC.
8. Girardin BW, et al. Color atlas of sexual assault. St Louis, MS, Mosby, 1997.
9. Burgess AW, Holmstrom LL. Rape trauma syndrome and post-traumatic stress response. In: Burgess AW, ed. Rape and sexual assault: a research handbook. New York, NY, Garland Publishing Inc., 1985:46–60.
10. Guidelines and protocols: Medico-legal care for survivors/victims of sexual violence: Ministry of Health and Family Welfare, Government of India, dated 19 March 2014, New Delhi.

Medical Examination and Reporting for Sexual Violence

Rajshree Dayanand Katke

Sexual violence is a significant cause of physical and psychological harm and suffering for women and children. Although sexual violence mostly affects women and girls, boys are also subject to child sexual abuse. Adult men, especially in police custody or prisons may also be subject to sexual violence, as also sexual minorities, especially the transgender community. Sexual violence takes various forms and the perpetrators range from strangers to state agencies to intimate partners; evidence shows that perpetrators are usually persons known to the survivor.

The World Health Organisation (WHO) defines sexual violence as "any sexual Act, attempt to obtain a sexual Act, unwanted sexual comments/advances and Acts to traffic, or otherwise directed against a person's sexuality, using coercion, threats of harm, or physical force, by any person regardless of relationship to the victim in any setting, including but not limited to home and work" (WHO, 2003).

The Ministry of Health and Family Welfare recognizes the critical role to be played by the health professionals and health systems in caring for survivors/victims of sexual violence and collecting relevant evidence so that the culprit could be brought to book.

Guidelines for Health Professionals (Figure 21.1)

The following guidelines are for health professionals when a survivor of sexual violence reports to a hospital[1]

   i. Initial resuscitation/first aid
  ii. Informed consent for examination, evidence collection, police procedures
 iii. Detailed history taking
 iv. Medical examination
  v. Age estimation (physical/dental/radiological), if requested by the investigating agency
 vi. Evidence collection as per the protocol
 vii. Documentation
viii. Packing, sealing and handing over the collected evidence to police
 ix. Treatment of injuries
  x. Testing/prophylaxis for STIs, HIV, hepatitis B and pregnancy
 xi. Psychological support and counseling
 xii. Referral for further help (shelter, legal support)

Documentation

Record the name of hospital where the survivor is being examined followed by the following:

   i. Name, address, age and sex (male/female/other) of the survivor

  ii. Date and time of receiving the patient in the hospital and commencement of examination

 iii. Name of the person who brought the survivor and relationship to accompanying persons

 iv. Informed consent: A survivor may approach a health facility under the circumstances:

- on his/her own only for treatment of effects of assault
- with a police requisition after police complaint or
- with a court directive

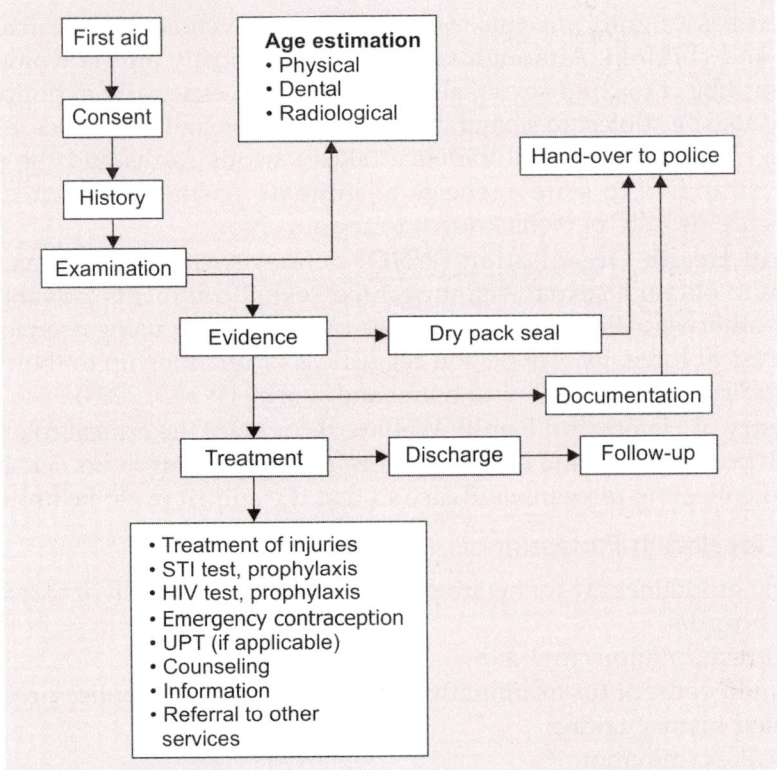

Figure 21.1: Guidelines for health professionals

If a person has come directly to the hospital without the police requisition, the hospital is bound to provide treatment and conduct a medical examination with consent of the survivor/parent/guardian (depending on age). A police requisition is not required for this.

If a person has come on his/her own without FIR, she/he may or may not want to lodge a complaint but requires a medical examination and treatment. Even in such cases the doctor is bound to inform the police as per law.

However, neither court nor police can force the survivor to undergo medical examination. It has to be with the informed consent of the survivor/parent/guardian (depending on the age).

In case the survivor does not want to pursue a police case, a MLC must be made and she must be informed that she has the right to refuse to file FIR. An informed refusal must be documented in such cases.

If the person has come with a police requisition or wishes to lodge a complaint later, the information about medico-legal case (MLC) no. and police station should be recorded.

Doctors are legally bound to examine and provide treatment to survivors of sexual violence. The timely reporting, documentation and collection of forensic evidence may assist the investigation of this crime. Police personnel should not be present during any part of the examination.

Only in situations, which are life-threatening the doctor may initiate treatment without consent as per **Section 92 of IPC**.

The consent form must be signed by the person himself/herself if he/she is above 12 years of age. Consent must be taken from the guardian/parent if the survivor is under the age of 12 years.

In case of persons with mental disability, his/her parent/guardian/any other person with whom the survivor is comfortable may be present.

Two marks of identification such as moles, scars, tattoos, etc. preferably from the exposed parts of the body should be documented. While describing identification mark emphasis should be on size, site, surface, shape, colour, fixity to underlying structures. Left thumb impression is to be taken in the space provided.

Relevant Medical/Surgical History

Menstrual history (cycle length and duration, date of last menstrual period) must be noted. If the survivor is menstruating at the time of examination then a second examination is required on a later date in order to record the injuries clearly. Some amount of evidence is lost because of menstruation. Hence, it is important to record whether the survivor was menstruating at the time of assault/examination.

Vaccination history is important with regard to tetanus and hepatitis B.

Sexual Violence History

Be sensitive to the survivor as she has experienced a traumatic episode and she/he may not be able to provide all the details. Explain to him/her that the process of history taking is important for further treatment and for filing a case if needed.

Create an environment of trust so that the survivor is able to speak out. Do not pass judgmental remarks.

- A relative could be present with the consent of the survivor, if she/he is comfortable.
- Details of the date, time and location of incident of sexual violence should be recorded. In case of more than one assailant, their number should be recorded along with the names and relation if known.
- Survivor or an informant may narrate the incident. If history is narrated by a person other than the survivor herself, his/her name should be noted. Especially if the identity of assailants is revealed it is better to also have a counter-signature of the informant.

General Physical Examination

- Record if the person is oriented in space and time and is able to respond to all the questions asked by the doctor. Any signs of intoxication by ingestion or injection of drug/alcohol must be noted.
- Pulse, BP, respiration temperature and state of pupils is recorded.
- A note is made of the state of clothing if it is the same as that worn at the time of assault. If it is freshly torn or has stains of blood/semen/mud, etc.; the site, size, and colour of stains should be described.

Examination for Injuries

- Presence of injuries is only observed in one-third cases of forced sexual intercourse. Absence of injuries does not mean the survivor has consented to sexual activity. As per law, if resistance was not offered that does not mean the person has consented.
- The entire body surface should be inspected carefully for signs of bruises, physical torture injuries, nail abrasions, teeth bite marks, cuts, lacerations, fracture, tenderness, any other injury, boils, lesions, discharge specially on the scalp, face, neck, shoulders, breast, wrists, forearms, medial aspect of upper arms, thighs and buttocks.
- Describe the type of injury (abrasion, laceration, incised, contusion, etc.), site, size, shape, colour, swelling, signs of healing, simple/grievous, dimensions. Mention possible weapon of infliction such as hard, blunt, rough, sharp.
- Injuries are best represented when marked on body charts. They must be numbered on the body chart and each must be described in detail.
- Describe any stains seen on the body—the type of stain (blood, semen, lubricant, etc.), its actual site, size and colour. Mention the number of swabs collected and their sites.

Local Examination of Genital Parts/Other Orifices

A. External genital area and perineum is observed carefully for evidence of injury, seminal stains and stray pubic hair. Pubic hair is examined for any seminal deposits/stray hair. Combing is done to pick up any stray hair or foreign material, and sample of pubic hair, and matted pubic hair is taken and preserved. If pubic hair is shaven, a note is made.

B. In case of female survivors, the vulva is inspected systematically for any signs of recent injury such as bleeding, tears, bruises, abrasions, swelling, or discharge and infection involving urethral meatus and vestibule, labia majora and minora, fourchette, introitus and hymen.

Examination of the vagina of an adult female is done with the help of a sterile speculum lubricated with warm saline/sterile water. Gentle retraction allows for inspection of the vaginal canal. Look for bruises, redness, bleeding and tears, which may even extend onto the perineum, especially in the case of very young girls.

- Toluidine blue is available it is sprayed and excess is wiped out. Micro injuries will stand out in blue. Care should be taken that all these tests are done only after swabs for trace evidence are collected.
- Per speculum examination is not a must in the case of children/young girls when there is no history of penetration and no visible injuries.

- Per vaginum examination commonly referred to by lay persons as 'two-finger test', must not be conducted for establishing rape/sexual violence and the size of the vaginal introitus has no bearing on a case of sexual violence. Per vaginum examination can be done only in adult women when medically indicated.

  A per speculum or per vaginal examination should be done only if needed for detection of injuries or for medical treatment. Record the reason why the per speculum or per vaginal examination is being done.
- The status of hymen is irrelevant because the hymen can be torn due to several reasons such as cycling, riding or masturbation among other things.
- An intact hymen does not rule out sexual violence, and a torn hymen does not prove previous sexual intercourse. **Hymen should therefore be treated like any other part of the genitals** while documenting examination findings in cases of sexual violence. Only those that are relevant to the episode of assault (findings such as fresh tears, bleeding, edema, etc.) are to be documented.
- Genital findings must also be marked on body charts and numbered accordingly.

C. Bleeding/swelling/tears/discharge/stains/warts around the anus and anal orifice must be documented.

Per rectal examination to detect tears/stains/fissures/hemorrhoids in the anal canal must be carried out and relevant swabs from these sites should be collected.

D. Oral cavity should also be examined for any evidence of bleeding, discharge, tear, edema, tenderness.

Sample Collection/Investigations for Hospital Laboratory/Clinical Laboratory

- Radiographs of the wrist, elbow, shoulders, dental examination, etc. can be advised for age estimation.
- For any suspected fracture/injury-appropriate investigation for the relevant part of the body is advised.
- Urine pregnancy test should be performed by the doctor on duty and the report should be entered.
- Blood is collected for evidence of baseline HIV status, VDRL and HBsAg.

Samples Collection for Central/State Forensic Science Laboratory

- **After assessment of the case, determine what evidence needs to be collected. It would depend upon the nature of the assault, time lapsed between assault and examination and if the person has bathed/washed herself since the assault.**
- If the woman reports **within 96 hours** of the assault, all evidence including swabs must be collected, based on the nature of the assault that has occurred. The likelihood of finding evidence after 72 hours is greatly reduced.
- The spermatozoa can be identified only for 72 hours after assault. So, if the survivor has suffered the assault more than three days ago, no need to take swabs for spermatozoa. In such cases swabs should only be sent for semen.
- The nature of the swabs taken is determined to a large extent by the history and nature of assault and time lapse between the incident and examination.
- **Request the survivor to stand on a large sheet of paper,** so as to collect any specimens of foreign material, e.g. grass, mud, pubic or scalp hair, etc. which may have been

left on the persons body from the site of assault or the accused. This sheet of paper is folded carefully and preserved in a bag to be sent to FSL for trace evidence detection.

- Clothes that the survivor was wearing at the time of the incident of sexual violence are of evidentiary value if there are any stains/tears/trace evidence on them. Hence, they must be preserved. Please describe each piece of clothing separately and with proper labeling. Presence of stains, semen, blood, foreign material, etc. should be properly noted. Also note if there are any tears or other marks on the clothes. If clothes were changed then the survivor must be asked for the clothes that were worn at the time of assault and these must be preserved.
- Always ensure that the clothes and samples are air-dried before storing them in their respective packets. Ensure that the clothing is folded in such a manner that the stained parts are not in contact with unstained parts of the clothing. Pack each piece of clothing in a separate bag, seal and label it duly.

Body Evidence

- Swabs are used to collect blood stains on the body, foreign material on the body surfaces, seminal stains on the skin surfaces and other stains.
- Detection of scalp hair and pubic hair of the accused on the survivor's body (and vice versa) has evidentiary value. Collect **loose** scalp and pubic hair by combing. **Intact** scalp and pubic hair is also collected from the survivor so that it can be matched with loose hair collected from the accused. All hair must be collected in the catchment paper which is then folded and sealed.
- If there is struggle during the sexual violence, with accused and survivor scratching each other, epithelial cells of one may be present under the nails of the other that can be used for DNA detection. **Nail clippings and scrapings must be taken for both hands and packed separately**. Ensure that there is no underlying tissue contamination while clipping nails.
- Blood is collected for grouping and also helps in matching blood stains at the scene of crime.
- Collect blood and urine for detection of drugs/alcohol as the influence of drugs/ alcohol has a bearing on the outcome of the entire investigation. If such substances are found in the blood, the validity of consent is called into question. In a given case, for instance, there may not be any physical or genital injuries. In such a situation, ascertaining the presence of drug/alcohol in the blood or urine is important since this may have affected the survivor's ability to resist. Urine sample may be collected in a container to test for drugs and alcohol levels.
- Venous blood is collected with a sterile syringe and needle provided and transferred to 3 sterile vials/vacutainers for the following purposes:
  - Plain vial—blood grouping and drug estimation
  - Sodium fluoride—alcohol estimation
  - EDTA—DNA analysis
- Collect oral swabs for detection of semen and spermatozoa. Oral swabs should be taken from the posterior parts of the buccal cavity, behind the last molars where the chances of finding any evidence are highest.

Genital and Anal Evidence

- In the case of any suspected seminal deposits on the pubic hair of the woman, collect matted portion of the pubic hair; allow drying in the shade and placing in an envelope.
- Pubic hair of the survivor is then combed for specimens of the offender's pubic hair. A comb must be used for this purpose and a catchment paper must be used to collect and preserve the specimens. Cuttings of the pubic hair are also taken for the purpose of comparison or to serve as control samples. If pubic hair has been shaved, do not fail to make a mention of it in the records.
- Take two swabs from the vulva, vagina, anal opening for ano-genital evidence. Swabs must be collected depending on the history and examination. Swabs from orifices must be collected only if there is a history of penetration.
  - Two vaginal smears are to be prepared on the glass slide provided, air-dried in the shade and sent for seminal fluid/spermatozoa examination.
  - Swab sticks for collecting samples should be moistened with distilled water provided
  - **Swabs must be air-dried, but nor dried in direct sunlight.**
  - While handing over the samples, a requisition letter addressed to the FSL, stating what all samples are being sent and what each sample needs to be tested for should be stated. For example, "vaginal swab to be tested for semen". This form must be signed by the examining doctor as well as the officer to whom the evidence is handed over.
  - Please ensure that the numbering of the individual packets is in keeping with the requisition form. FSL samples will not be received unless they are packed separately, sealed, labeled and handed over.

Provisional Clinical Opinion (Table 21.1)

- Drafting of provisional opinion should be done immediately after examination of the survivor **on the basis of history and findings of detailed clinical examination of the survivor**.
- The provisional opinion must, in brief, mention relevant aspects of the history of sexual violence, clinical findings and samples which are sent for analysis to FSL.
- **An inference must be drawn in the opinion**, correlating the history and clinical findings.

It should always be kept in mind that normal examination findings neither refute nor confirm the forceful sexual intercourse. Hence, circumstantial/other evidence may please be taken into consideration.

Absence of injuries or negative laboratory results may be due to

A. Instability of survivor to offer resistance to the assailant because of intoxication or threats

B. Delay in reporting for examination

C. Activities such as urinating, washing, bathing, changing clothes or douching which may lead to loss of evidence

D. Use of condom/vasectomy or diseases of vas

This reasoning must be mentioned while formulating the opinion (Tables 21.1 to 21.3).

Genital injuries	Physical injuries	Opinion	Rationale why forced penetrative sex cannot be ruled out	What can FSL detect
Table 21.1: Provisional opinion				
Present	Present	There are signs s/o recent use of force/forceful penetration of vagina/anus. Sexual violence cannot be ruled out	Evidence of semen/spermatozoa are yet to be tested by laboratory examination in case of penile penetration	Evidence of semen except when condom was used
Present	Absent	There are signs s/o recent force-ful penetration of vagina/anus	Evidence of semen/spermatozoa are yet to be tested in case of penile penetration. The lack of physical injuries could be because of the survivor being unconscious, under the effect of alcohol/drugs, overpowered or threatened. It could be because there was fingering or penetration by object with or without use of lubricant, which is an offence under Section 375 of IPC	Evidence of semen/lubricant except when condom was used
Absent	Present	There are signs of use of force; however, vaginal or anal or oral penetration cannot be ruled out	The lack of injuries could be because of the survivor being unconscious, under the effect of alcohol/drugs, overpowered or threatened	Evidence of semen/lubricant
Absent	Absent	There are no signs of use of force; however, final opinion is reserved pending availability of FSL reports. Sexual violence cannot be ruled out	The lack of genital injuries could be because of use of lubricant. The lack of physical injuries could be because of the survivor being unconscious, under the effect of alcohol/drugs, over-powered or threatened. It could also be because there was fingering or penetration by an object with use of lubricant, which is an offence under Section 375 of IPC	Evidence of semen, lubricant and drug/alcohol

Final opinion: To be formulated after receiving reports from the FSL.

Table 21.2: Final opinion

Sr. No.	Genital injuries	Physical injuries/ diseases	FSL report injuries/diseases	Final opinion
For penile penetration				
1.	Present	Present	Positive for presence of semen	There are signs s/o forceful vaginal/anal intercourse
2.	Present	Absent	Positive for presence of semen	There are signs s/o forceful vaginal/anal intercourse
3.	Absent	Present	Positive for presence of semen	There are signs s/o forceful vaginal/anal intercourse
4.	Absent	Absent	Positive for presence of semen	There are signs s/o vaginal/anal intercourse
5.	Absent	Absent	Positive for drugs/alcohol and semen	There are signs s/o vaginal/anal intercourse under the influence of drugs/alcohol
For non-penile penetration				
6.	Present	Present	FSL report is negative for semen/alcohol/drugs/lubricant	There are no signs s/o vaginal/anal intercourse, but there is e/o physical and genital assault
7.	Present	Absent	FSL report is negative for semen/alcohol/drugs/lubricant	There are no signs s/o vaginal/anal intercourse, but there is e/o genital assault
8.	Absent	Present	FSL report is negative for semen/alcohol/drugs/lubricant	There are no signs s/o vaginal/anal intercourse, but there is e/o physical assault
9.	Absent	Absent	FSL report is negative for semen/alcohol/drugs/lubricant	There are no signs suggestive of penetration of vagina/anus
10.	Absent	Absent	FSL report is positive for presence of lubricant only	There is a possibility of vaginal/anal penetration by lubricated object

Table 21.3: Opinion for non-penetrative assault

1. Bite marks present and/or FSL detects salivary stains	There are signs suggestive of evidence of bite mark/s on _____ site (time the injury)
2. Sucking marks (discoid, subcutaneous extravasation of blood, with or without bite marks) present and/or FSL detects salivary stains	There are signs suggestive of sucking mark/s on _____ site (time the injury)
3. Forceful fondling, with presence of bruises or contusions with or without fingernail marks	There are signs suggestive of forceful physical injuries on _____ site (time the injury) (which may be due to fondling)
4. Only forceful kissing and FSL detects salivary stains	There are signs suggestive of salivary contact (which may be due to kissing)

(Contd.)

Table 21.3: Opinion for non-penetrative assault (*Contd.*)	
5. If the history suggests forced masturbation by the assailant on the survivor and if there is evidence of seminal stains detected on the hands	There are signs suggestive on the survivor of seminal fluid contact (which may be due to masturbation)
6. In case there are no signs of sucking, licking detected, but the history suggests some such form of assault	It is still important to document a good history because the survivor may have had a bath or washed himself/herself.

REFERENCE

1. The presentation is compiled from the "Guidelines & Protocols, Medico-legal care for survivors/victims of Sexual Violence" issued by the Ministry of Health and Family Welfare downloaded from www.cehat.org>uploads>Publications>R83Manual.

Safe Kit and Formulating of Opinion and Diagnosis

Rashmi Jalvee

Abstract

Examining a survivor of sexual violence is a medico-legal emergency. There must be no delay in conducting an examination and collecting evidence. The history taking and examination should be carried out in complete privacy in the separate room set up in the hospital for examination. The Sexual Assault Forensic Evidence (SAFE) kit is used which contains all the requisite items for collecting and preserving physical evidence following a sexual violence: Once history taking and examination is done and evidence is collected, a provisional opinion is drafted. Normal examination findings neither refute nor confirm the forceful sexual intercourse. Hence, circumstantial/other evidence must be taken into consideration.

Article

Every hospital must have a standard operating procedure (SOP) for management of cases of sexual violence:
1. To provide comprehensive services.
2. For the smooth handling of the cases and clarity of roles of each staff.
3. To have uniform practice across all doctors in the hospital.

The SOP must be printed and available to all staff of the hospital.

Any registered medical practitioner can conduct examination and it is not mandatory for a gynaecologist to examine such a case. In case of a girl or woman, every possible effort should be made to find a female doctor but absence of availability of lady doctor, we should not deny or delay the treatment and examination. In case a female doctor is not available for the examination of a female survivor, a male doctor should conduct the examination in the presence of a female attendant. In case of a minor/person with disability, his/her parent/guardian/any other person with whom the survivor is comfortable may be present. Police personnel must not be allowed in the examination room during the consultation with the survivor. If the survivor requests, her relative may be present while the examination is done.

There must be no delay in conducting an examination and collecting evidence.

Providing treatment and necessary medical investigations is the prime responsibility of the examining doctor. Admission, evidence collection or filing a police complaint is not mandatory for providing treatment.

The history taking and examination should be carried out in complete privacy in the special room set up in the hospital for examination of sexual violence survivor. The room should have adequate space, sufficient lighting, a comfortable examination table, all the equipment required for a thorough examination, and the Sexual Assault Forensic Evidence (SAFE) kit containing the following items for collecting and preserving physical evidence following a sexual violence:

- Forms for documentation
- Large sheet of paper to undress over
- Paper bags for clothing collection
- Catchment paper
- Sterile cotton swabs and swab guards for biological evidence collection
- Comb
- Nail cutter
- Wooden stick for fingernail scrapings
- Small scissors
- Urine sample container
- Tubes/vials/vaccutainers for blood samples [ethylene diamine tetra-acetic acid (EDTA), plain, sodium fluoride]
- Syringes and needle for drawing blood
- Distilled water
- Disposable gloves
- Glass slides
- Envelopes or boxes for individual evidence samples
- Labels
- Lac (sealing wax) stick for sealing
- Clean clothing, shower/hygiene items for survivors use after the examination.

Other items for a forensic/medical examination and treatment that may be included are:

- Wood's lamp/good torch
- Vaginal speculums
- Drying rack for wet swabs and/or clothing
- Patient gown, cover sheet, blanket, pillow
- Post: It notes to collect trace evidence
- Camera (35 mm, digital with colour printer)
- Microscope
- Colposcope/magnifying glass
- Toluidine blue dye
- 1% acetic acid diluted spray
- Urine pregnancy test kit
- Surgilube (lubricating jelly)
- Medications

The collected samples for evidence may be preserved in the hospital till such time that police are able to complete their paperwork for dispatch to forensic lab test including DNA test samples.

After the examination is complete the survivor should be permitted to wash up, using the toiletries and the clothing provided by the hospital if her own clothing is taken as evidence.

Admission should not be insisted upon unless the survivor requires indoor stay for observation/treatment.

Survivors of sexual violence should receive all services completely free of cost. This includes OPD/inpatient registration, lab and radiology investigations, urine pregnancy test (UPT) and medicines. The casualty medical officer must label the case papers for any sexual violence case as "free" so that free treatment is ensured. Medicines should be prescribed from those available in the hospital. If certain investigations or medicines are not available, the social worker at the hospital should ensure that the survivor is compensated for investigations/medicines from outside.

A copy of all documentation (including that pertaining to medico-legal examination and treatment) must be provided to the survivor free of cost.

The following guidelines are for health professionals when a survivor of sexual violence reports to a hospital. The guidelines describe in detail the stepwise approach to be used for a comprehensive response to the sexual violence survivor as follows:

  i. Initial resuscitation/first aid
 ii. Informed consent for examination, evidence collection, police procedures
iii. Detailed history taking
 iv. Medical examination
  v. Age estimation (physical/dental/radiological), if requested by the investigating agency.
 vi. Evidence collection as per the protocol
vii. Documentation
viii. Packing, sealing and handing over the collected evidence to police
 ix. Treatment of injuries
  x. Testing/prophylaxis for STIs, HIV, hepatitis B and pregnancy
 xi. Psychological support and counselling
xii. Referral for further help (shelter, legal support)

Provisional Clinical Opinion (Table 22.1)

- Drafting of provisional opinion should be done immediately after examination of the survivor based on history and findings of detailed clinical examination of the survivor.
- The provisional opinion must, in brief, mention relevant aspects of the history of sexual violence, clinical findings and samples which are sent for analysis to FSL.
- An inference must be drawn in the opinion, correlating the history and clinical findings.

The following section offers some scenarios about ways to draft a provisional and final opinion. However, this list is not exhaustive, and readers are advised to form provisional opinions based on the examples given below.

It should be always kept in mind that normal examination findings neither refute nor confirm the forceful sexual intercourse. Hence, circumstantial/other evidence may please be taken into consideration.

Absence of injuries or negative laboratory results may be due to:
- Inability of survivor to offer resistance to the assailant because of intoxication or threats

- Delay in reporting for examination
- Activities such as urinating, washing, bathing, changing clothes or douching which may lead to loss of evidence.
- Use of condom/vasectomy or diseases of vas.

This reasoning must be mentioned while formulating the opinion (Tables 22.1 to 22.3).

Table 22.1: Provisional opinion				
Genital injuries	Physical injuries	Opinion	Rationale why forced penetrative sex cannot be ruled out	What can FSL detect
Present	Present	There are signs s/o recent use of force/forceful penetration of vagina/anus. Sexual violence cannot be ruled out	Evidence of semen/spermatozoa are yet to be tested by laboratory examination in case of penile penetration	Evidence of semen except when condom was used
Present	Absent	There are signs s/o recent force-ful penetration of vagina/anus	Evidence of semen/spermatozoa are yet to be tested in case of penile penetration. The lack of physical injuries could be because of the survivor being unconscious, under the effect of alcohol/drugs, overpowered or threatened. It could be because there was fingering or penetration by object with or without use of lubricant, which is an offence under Section 375 of IPC	Evidence of semen/lubricant except when condom was used
Absent	Present	There are signs of use of force; however, vaginal or anal or oral penetration cannot be ruled out	The lack of injuries could be because of the survivor being unconscious, under the effect of alcohol/drugs, overpowered or threatened	Evidence of semen/lubricant
Absent	Absent	There are no signs of use of force; however, final opinion is reserved pending availability of FSL reports. Sexual violence cannot be ruled out	The lack of genital injuries could be because of use of lubricant. The lack of physical injuries could be because of the survivor being unconscious, under the effect of alcohol/drugs, over-powered or threatened. It could also be because there was fingering or penetration by an object with use of lubricant, which is an offence under Section 375 of IPC	Evidence of semen, lubricant and drug/alcohol

Final opinion: To be formulated after receiving reports from the FSL.

Table 22.2: Final opinion

Sr. No.	Genital injuries	Physical injuries/ diseases	FSL report injuries/diseases	Final opinion
For penile penetration				
1.	Present	Present	Positive for presence of semen	There are signs s/o forceful vaginal/anal intercourse
2.	Present	Absent	Positive for presence of semen	There are signs s/o forceful vaginal/anal intercourse
3.	Absent	Present	Positive for presence of semen	There are signs s/o forceful vaginal/anal intercourse
4.	Absent	Absent	Positive for presence of semen	There are signs s/o vaginal/ anal intercourse
5.	Absent	Absent	Positive for drugs/alcohol and semen	There are signs s/o vaginal/ anal intercourse under the influence of drugs/alcohol
For non-penile penetration				
6.	Present	Present	FSL report is negative for semen/alcohol/drugs/lubricant	There are no signs s/o vaginal/anal intercourse, but there is e/o physical and genital assault
7.	Present	Absent	FSL report is negative for semen/alcohol/drugs/lubricant	There are no signs s/o vaginal/anal intercourse, but there is e/o genital assault
8.	Absent	Present	FSL report is negative for semen/alcohol/drugs/lubricant	There are no signs s/o vaginal/anal intercourse, but there is e/o physical assault
9.	Absent	Absent	FSL report is negative for semen/alcohol/drugs/lubricant	There are no signs suggestive of penetration of vagina/ anus
10.	Absent	Absent	FSL report is positive for presence of lubricant only	There is a possibility of vaginal/anal penetration by lubricated object

Table 22.3: Opinion for non-penetrative assault

1. Bite marks present and/or FSL detects salivary stains	There are signs suggestive of evidence of bite mark/s on _____ site (time the injury)
2. Sucking marks (discoid, subcutaneous extravasation of blood, with or without bite marks) present and/or FSL detects salivary stains	There are signs suggestive of sucking mark/s on _____ site (time the injury)
3. Forceful fondling, with presence of bruises or contusions with or without fingernail marks	There are signs suggestive of forceful physical injuries on _____ site (time the injury) (which may be due to fondling)
4. Only forceful kissing and FSL detects salivary stains	There are signs suggestive of salivary contact (which may be due to kissing)

(Contd.)

Table 22.3: **Opinion for non-penetrative assault** *(Contd.)*

5. If the history suggests forced masturbation by the assailant on the survivor and if there is evidence of seminal stains detected on the hands	There are signs suggestive on the survivor of seminal fluid contact (which may be due to masturbation)
6. In case there are no signs of sucking, licking detected, but the history suggests some such form of assault	It is still important to document a good history because the survivor may have had a bath or washed him/herself.

CONCLUSION

With a lot of changes in the laws over the past few years, adequate dissemination of this information to all stakeholders of the health care sector along with proper training is required. This will help the survivors in bringing the perpetrators to book.

REFERENCE

1. The presentation is compiled from the "Guidelines and Protocols, medico-legal care for survivors/victims of Sexual Violence" issued by the Ministry of Health and Family Welfare downloaded from www.cehat.org>uploads>Publications>R83Manual.

Tips to Survive and be Safe for a Victim of Violence

Bhavini Shah Balakrishnan

#MeToo was a globe wide and the biggest anti-sexual abuse and anti-sexual harrasment movement initiated by a sexual harrassment survivor herself and an activist Tarana Burke.

Basic tips to be safe for a victim of violence of any form are listed below:

1. Choose a safe place to go in an emergency. It could be any place, a relative's house, a friend's house or a safe home.
2. Keep a trusted friend and a close neighbour in the loop always for help. Their job role would be:
   - Have a code word decided with neighbours and friends to alert them to call for help
   - Take children away from the house as soon as they sense a problem
   - Help keep a rescue bag with important keys and documents for emergency exit.
   - Have a list of important phone numbers and addresses in place.
3. Teach your children about their safety.
   - Teach the children to be alert and train them what to do if they sense danger.
   - Their job is to be safe and not to protect you.
   - They should know whom to call for help.
   - The escape route has to be rehearsed with them if they can maintain secrecy.
4. Put all sharps, guns and knives out of sight.
5. During a fight or emergency, stay out of rooms and areas from which it might be difficult to escape or get help.
   - Kitchen and garage—risk of injury
   - Bathroom—risk of getting locked and no escape
6. Gathering the most important documents, keys, benefit cards and emergency funds and put them in one place that is easily accesible.
7. Take only the important things when leaving. A police can escort you later to get your belongings.
8. Keep a bunch of keys and some money outside the house.
9. Rehearse the escape plan thoroughly including what doors or windows to be used, etc.

10. Keep your cell phone charged and with you at all times.
11. Document the abuse everytime by taking pictures of the bruises and injuries. Tell the doctor and get the copies of the medical record.
12. Learn skills that will help you be emotionally and financially independent. Look for a job. Start banking yourself. Learn to drive.

List of Important Documents to Carry when Leaving

- Passport
- Birth certificate
- Social security documents
- Bank documents and cheque books
- Bank cards
- Divorce and custody documents
- Important contact details of friends and family
- Important keys
- Comfort clothing for self and children
- Important medications
- Cell phone charger

Precautions to be taken if the Abuser is not Staying with the Victim or has been Removed from the House

1. Make sure to change the locks of the doors and windows.
2. Install peep holes in all the doors.
3. All doors should be grilled.
4. Definitely have CCTV cameras installed in the house and workplace.
5. Have a phone with caller ID.
6. Change the daily routine routes, super markets, child's day care, etc.
7. Inform the school and day care about the changes and who will pick the child, etc.

Case Discussions, Long-term Issues and Future Direction

Long-term Sequelae: VAW and US

Reena J Wani, Sachin Paprikar

Askios (a Greek word meaning "shadowless").
"Those of us with childhood wounds have many shadows that follow us into adulthood and prevent us from reaching our full potential. Through Askios, I hope to build a safe, supportive environment that frees us from our sense of isolation, enables us to develop coping skills, share our pain and our strengths, and move forward from the childhood experiences that have held us hostage so long."

askios.tripod.com was a website started by my childhood friend as an adult, who opened up many years later about the sexual abuse she faced as a child from an older cousin. Her pain and issues that came up during her adult life have been a stark reminder of the long-term effects that we as health care providers need to be aware of.

Sexual violence is a human rights issue, which violates the notion that victims are human beings *'born free and equal in dignity and rights'* (*Article One of the Universal Declaration of Human Rights*). Among other rights violations, sexual violence transgresses the right of victim/survivors to enjoy the highest attainable standard of physical and mental health.

But unfortunately sexual violence is a reality for millions of people worldwide and for women in particular. Global estimates published by WHO indicate that about 1 in 3 (35%) of women worldwide have experienced either physical and/or sexual intimate partner violence or non-partner sexual violence in their lifetime.[1]

Data on sexual violence typically come from police, clinical settings, nongovernmental organizations and survey research. The data collected and the global magnitude of the problem of sexual violence may be viewed as corresponding to an iceberg floating in water (Figure 24.1). Available data are drawn from different populations using a variety of measures of sexual violence and data accuracy is affected by nonreporting (Lievore, 2003).[2] The true prevalence of the many forms of sexual violence against girls and women is not known.

Health care providers (HCPs) have a large role to play in supporting the victims/survivors of sexual assault—medically, psychologically and in collecting evidence to assist prosecutions. For HCPs to play this role effectively they need an in-depth knowledge and skills that are necessary for the management of victims of sexual violence.

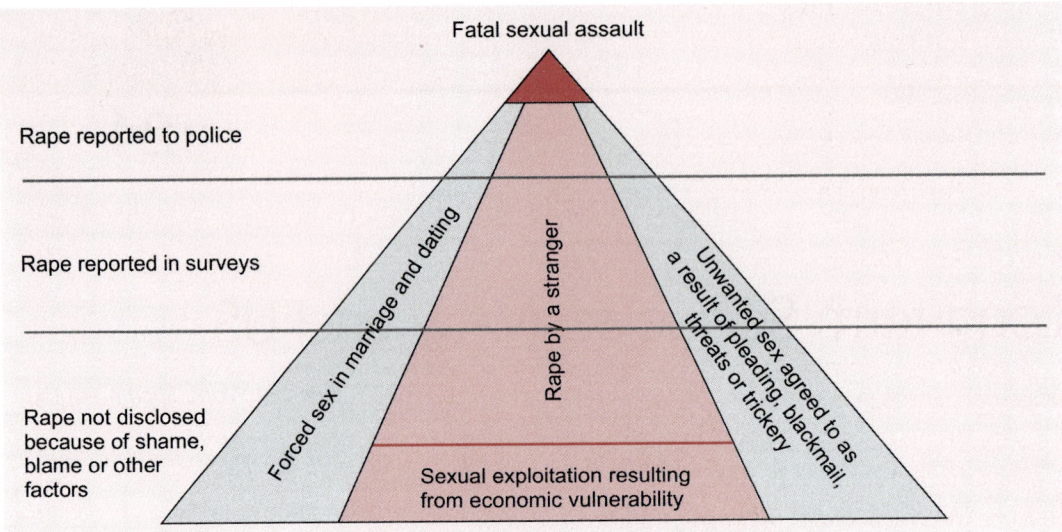

Figure 24.1: Tip of the Iceberg: Spectrum of violence against women

PRESENTATION

Could be in different ways to the health care system
- **Sexual disorders**
- **Psychosocial issues**
- **Need for counselling**
- **Self-abuse**
- **Personality disorders**

Case 1: Adult survivor of CSA: This childhood friend of mine was always smiling and jocular on the surface, but had many classic manifestations of the long-term issues, which was realized later in life as she opened up about the past, sought counseling and help.
- **Academic issues:** Difficulty in sticking to a particular subject/course in college, dropping out of chosen curriculum due to personal problems of adjustment.
- **Maintaining or establishing adult relationships often difficult:** Getting into short-term affairs with unsuitable/unstable candidates, not being able to sustain commitment.
- **Drug addiction, substance abuse:** Alcohol, weed, psychotropic drugs are used as a means of forgetting the past, or to escape the troubled mind. This snowballs into a vicious cycle of self-destruction.

Case 2: Sexual dysfunction and failure to consummate marriage: We have come across quite a few cases in our gynecological practice where sexual problems between the couple are causing marital difficulties, even leading to divorce. Some of them are deep-rooted in the past, and history of abuse should be gently but specifically explored and asked about, confidentially.
- **Vaginismus:** Involuntary spasms and contraction of the vagina may have an organic basis but can be due to fear/psychological impact of CSA as seen in some cases.

- **Frigidity/lack of libido:** It has been said somewhat crudely, "sex is not between the legs, but between the ears"—it is the interplay of emotions and attraction, mental state and psychological factors which can impact a relationship between 2 partners. It has been found that past negative experiences impact the psyche of survivors and can discolor their perception of this biological part of a relationship.

Case 3: Suicide: This is another sad story seen by us in real life, RW was called to assess

- **Resident doctor with drug overdose, admitted to MICU**
- **History of failed relationships, was recently married, gold medalist in PG**
- **History of CSA by uncle for many years, unresolved conflicts** was revealed by her teacher later, who had tried to encourage her to seek help.

India recorded an average of 87 rape cases daily in 2019 and overall 4,05,861 cases of crime against women during the year, a rise of over 7% from 2018.[3] According to National Crime Records Bureau 30641 cases of rape were registered in India in 2019.[3] According to National Family Health Survey 4 (NFHS-4), the prevalence of lifetime physical and/or sexual intimate partner violence is 28.8% while the prevalence of physical and/or sexual intimate partner violence in the last 12 months is 22%.[4]

PSYCHOLOGICAL HEALTH CONSEQUENCES

Why did the Bollywood child star *Daisy Irani* choose to speak up at age 67 years, to media about the childhood sexual abuse she faced at age 5 years from the man deputed by her parents to "protect" her on outstation shooting trips? This is a classic example of the baggage that survivors carry down the years, which weighs them down and should be shed off at the earliest possible.

Rape trauma syndrome (RTS)[5] is a common reaction to rape or sexual assault. Three phases have been described:

  i. *Acute*, which occurs immediately after the assault.
  ii. *Outward adjustment phase*, during which the individual resumes his or her life but inside is suffering from considerable turmoil.
  iii. *Resolution phase*, during which the individual realises though he or she may never forget the assault it is no more a central focus of their lives.

This assumes that individuals will take steps forward and backwards in their healing process and that while there are phases it is not a linear progression and will be different for every person. RTS is now recognized as a type of post-traumatic stress disorder (PTSD).

Short-term psychological effects seen are[6, 7]
- Fear and shock
- Physical and emotional
- Pain
- Powerlessness
- Intense self-disgust
- Worthlessness
- Apathy
- Denial

- Numbing
- Withdrawal
- An inability to function normally in their daily lives.

Long-term psychological effects seen are[6,7]

- Depression and chronic anxiety
- Feelings of vulnerability
- Loss of control
- Loss of self-esteem
- Emotional distress
- Impaired sense of self
- Nightmares
- Self-blame
- Mistrust
- Avoidance and post-traumatic stress disorder
- Chronic mental disorders
- Committing suicide or endangering their lives.

Choices? Way Forward?

"Cure sometimes, relieve often and comfort always" is a mantra that we can follow as health care providers, and our approach and initial response to possible Acts of violence can impact the future life of survivors.

Psychological Counselling

- Most victims find counselling helpful in recovering and moving on.
- Follow-up sessions for counselling are equally important.
- If mental health professionals or crisis counselors are available that is ideal.
- But lack of such a person is not an excuse "that as a doctor my primary responsibility is the medical examination and medico-legal aspects and I have not time for this".
- Every physician dealing with sexual assault survivors need to learn basic counseling skills.

The literature has widely recognized the importance of two important areas when counseling survivors of sexual assault: *Acute post-sexual assault needs and its enduring effects*.

First Step—Build a Rapport!

- Appreciate the survivor's strength in coming to the hospital as it requires courage to overcome several barriers.
- Never say or do anything to suggest disbelief regarding the incident.
- Do not pass judgmental remarks or comments that might appear unsympathetic.
- Addressing survivor's emotional well-being, recognize that survivors may present varied emotions.
- Encourage the survivor to express her feelings, *to speak of the unspeakable*.
- Encourage survivors to seek crisis counseling.

- Assess for suicidal ideation.
- Make a safety assessment and safety plan.
- Involve family and friends in healing process of survivor.
- Create an enabling atmosphere, establishing trust.
- Speak to survivor in a private space, *ask alone and ask safely*.
- Do not label non-reporting to police as false case.
- Assure the survivor that her treatment will not be compromised.
- Inform survivor of available resources, referrals, legal rights so that she can take an informed decision.

Post-trauma Feelings

- Most survivors may not openly express their feelings.
- It is important to explain to them the range of feelings that they may experience such as sleeplessness, anxiety, nervousness, crying spells, feelings of ending one's life, anger and flashbacks (RTS, emotional reactions post-rape) after an assault.
- It must also be discussed that such reactions are normal after a traumatic episode and professional help should be taken.

Crisis Counseling can Help in Overcoming Trauma

- Explaining to survivors that
  - *"Rape" is a violation of bodily integrity and not a loss of honor, modesty or chastity but a violation of his/her rights"*;
  - *Assault is an abuse of power and not an Act of lust;*
- Positive messaging such as *"you are not responsible for rape"*, *"It is not about the clothes you wear"*.
- Convey important messages such as: The survivor is not responsible for precipitating the Act of rape by any of her actions or inactions.

Any incident of sexual violence leads to a feeling of powerlessness amongst survivors. This counseling would enable the survivor to discard the feelings of self-blame, as it is the perpetrator who should feel ashamed about the Act, and help in rebuilding survivor's confidence in self.

Helping Survivors to Prepare for Medical Examination

- It is important to recognize the covert feelings and explain the purpose of medical examination.
- Explaining the purpose of internal examination and steps in conducting it can help survivors to make sense of what is happening to them.
- This can help in regaining control over the situation.
- While making referrals providers must ensure confidentiality and privacy of survivors so that they are not embarrassed due to being identified as a 'survivor of sexual violence'.

Facilitating Medical Procedures

- Ensure confidentiality and explain to the survivor that she/he must reveal the entire history to health professional without fear.

- Explain to the survivor in simple and understandable language, the rationale for various procedures, details of how they will be performed.
- The survivor may be persuaded not to hide anything.

Do's and Don'ts

- Support that responds to her concerns, but does not intrude.
- Ensure confidentiality, but inform the limits.
- Asking about her history of violence, listening carefully, but not pressuring her to talk.
- Care should be taken when discussing sensitive topics when interpreters are involved.
- Assisting her to increase safety for herself and her children, where needed providing or mobilizing social support.

Heal the World[8]

People from across the world come together to mark **International Day for Elimination of Violence Against Women (VAW)** which was started by the United Nations General Assembly on 25th November 2012. This day of global importance is followed by 16 days of Activism culminating in Human Rights Day on **10th December, World Human Rights Day**. People wear **orange** to take a positive stand against violence and WHO launches new manual to strengthen the health system for better survival of women survival of violence. The UN System's 16 Days of Activism against Gender-based Violence activities, from 25th Nov to 10th Dec 2020 took place under the 2020 global theme: *"Orange the World: Fund, Respond, Prevent, Collect!"*.

We organized a series of events nationally and locally, including posters/slogan and skit competitions, and launched a booklet "KAVACH" on FOGSI website with helpline numbers for women and girls.[10]

Interventions[11, 12]

Health service providers have a particular responsibility *to identify, understand and ameliorate the harmful health effects of sexual violence*. Supportive services can minimize all forms of harm experienced by the victim/survivor. These include the long-term physical and psychological effects associated with rape and sexual assault, many of which are likely to compound in the absence of an appropriate and timely response.

Reporting or disclosure of sexual violence gives HCPs an important opportunity to provide competent, compassionate, and appropriate care to victim/survivors and hereby start the process of recovery.[9] Currently, most of these interventions are therapeutic or counselling interventions. To be meaningful, these interventions must respond to survivors' needs and concerns, *individually*.

Though the main focus of mental health interventions has been the treatment of the mental health consequences of sexual violence, it is important to note victims of sexual assault may experience forms of psychological distress that do not meet the usual criteria for the diagnosis of psychological disorders.

The literature identifies two main psychotherapeutic approaches in relation to the treatment of victims of sexual assault: Cognitive therapies and feminist (or group) therapies.

Cognitive therapies include: Cognitive behaviour therapy, rational emotive therapy and cognitive processing therapy. The goal of therapy is to change psychological distress by challenging and changing the distorted cognitions which give rise to it, based on the assumption that psychological distress and behavioural dysfunction can be produced by inaccurate and dysfunctional thinking.

Cognitive behavioural therapy (CBT) involves a number of different techniques, such as exposure to traumatic memories, cognitive restructuring and eye movement desensitization and reprocessing.

Feminist therapy helps the survivor/victim understand that such violence is a societal problem not just an individual problem and that sexual violence is reinforced by gender-based differences in privilege and power that play out within interpersonal relationships.

CONCLUSION

Just as sexual violence results from the complex interplay of individuals, relationships, social-cultural factors, the solution must also involve all those who have the opportunity to reduce such violence and eliminate its preventable harms by working together

- *Increasing the awareness of the law, collaboration with NGOs, provision of services under one roof.*
- *Involvement of different organizations in this issue.*
- *Streamlining services and training health care workers are the way forward.*
- *A broader understanding of the nature of sexual assault can assist health practitioners to more effectively recognize and respond to the presenting needs of survivors and their loved ones.*

REFERENCES

1. Violence against women [Internet]. Who.int. 2021 [cited 24 January 2021]. Available from: https://www.who.int/news-room/fact-sheets/detail/violence-against-women#: ~:text = Global % 20 estimates % 20 published % 20 by % 20 WHO, violence % 20 is % 20 intimate % 20 partner % 20 violence.

2. Nonreporting and hidden recording of sexual assault in Australia. Canberra: Australian Institute of Criminology. [Internet]. Lievore, D. 2003. [cited 24 January 2021]. Available from: https://www.aic.gov.au/publications/tandi/tandi359

3. Crime in India 2019 | National Crime Records Bureau [Internet]. Ncrb.gov.in. 2021 [cited 24 January 2021]. Available from: https://ncrb.gov.in/en/crime-india-2019-0

4. National Family Health Survey [Internet]. Rchiips.org. 2021 [cited 24 January 2021]. Available from: http://rchiips.org/nfhs/#

5. Rape Trauma Syndrome [Internet]. rainn.org. 2008 [cited 24 January 2021]. Available from: https://apps.rainn.org

6. Manual for Medical Examination of Sexual Assault [Internet]. Cehat.org. 2010 [cited 24 January 2021]. Available from: http://www.cehat.org/go/uploads/Publications/R83Manual.pdf.

7. Guidelines and Protocols, medico-legal care for survivors/victims of sexual violence [Internet]. Main.mohfw.gov.in. 2013 [cited 24 January 2021]. Available from: https://main.mohfw.gov.in/sites/default/files/953522324.pdf

8. Strengthening the health system response to violence against women [Internet]. World Health Organization. 2021 [cited 24 January 2021]. Available from: https://www.who.int/reproductive

health/topics/violence/internationalday/en/#:~:text = 25th % 20 November % 202016% 3A% 20 Every%20year,Day%20on%20the%2010th%20December.

9. Sexual Assault [Internet]. Acog.org. 2019 [cited 24 January 2021]. Available from: https://www.acog.org/clinical/clinical-guidance/committee-opinion/articles/2019/04/sexual-assault

10. KAVACH Booklet for Women Safety. A burning issue: The Federation of Obstetric and Gynecological Societies of India [Internet]. https://www.fogsi.org/. 2020 [cited 24 January 2021]. Available from: https://www.fogsi.org/kavach-booklet-for-women-safety-a-burning-issue/

11. Services for victim/ survivors of sexual assault identifying needs, interventions and provision of services in Australia [Internet]. Aifs.gov.au. 2006 [cited 24 January 2021]. Available from: https://aifs.gov.au/sites/default/files/publication-documents/acssa_issues6.pdf

12. Corey G. Theory and Practice of Counseling and Psychotherapy. 7th ed. Thomson: Brooks Cole; 2005.

Psychosocial Care for Violence Survivors

Bhavini Shah Balakrishnan

Around the world, one in every three women is beaten, coerced into sex or abused in some or the other way and most often by someone she knows.

Domestic violence is one of the most serious and most common forms of violence against women yet always pushed under the carpet. The fact that surprises us the most is that domestic violence is prevalent in all societies and culture. The consequences of violence poses a risk to victims' physical as well as mental health and also the quality of their life, both private and professional.

Post-traumatic stress disorders (PTSDs) are often high, especially in victims who have experienced multiple assaults. The cumulative effect of sexual violence may result in increased rates of alcohol and drug abuse, depression, and suicidal behavior. Immediately after rape or other assaults, victims can experience shock, intense fear, numbness, confusion, feeling of helplessness, in addition to self blame and high levels of anxiety.

While specific guidelines, protocols, or implementation strategies may vary, the management and provision of health care to victims should include the following procedures: Physical documentation and patient history, medical treatment, collection of forensic evidence, and psychosocial care.

Often the psychological needs of victims of sexual violence are overlooked, even in settings that offer medical services and have the facility for psychological care.

Before beginning any form of psychosocial treatment, it is important to identify the type of disorder the victim suffers. It was believed for many years that the most common disorder associated with sexual violence was post-traumatic stress disorder (PTSD). In reality, depression and anxiety are more common outcomes, even long after the event.

When we wish to focus on the psychosocial care of the survivors, the most important thing is to connect with them in a way that they get comfortable, talking about their pain. Leaving an abusive relationship is probably one of the toughest choices to make. Appropriate support thus plays a crucial role. A few important steps we need to follow are:

Step 1: To identify and establish contact

Victims are employing different survival strategies in order to protect themselves and their children from the abuser. There is no uniform approach but there are certain guidelines that should be followed.

You need to find that right connection with whoever that person is. Not everyone is going to connect with everyone. Always remember to be patient, non-judgmental, and compassionate.

Make sure the right questions are asked; questions targetting the victims, behaviour, etc. should be avoided.

A safe and trusted environment needs to be provided with full confidentiality maintained.

Ask yourself a simple question: "Is it safe to ask about violence?"

Explain the victim that her safety is a priority. Therefore, it is important to report violence, get help and be safe.

Explain to her that confidentiality is maintained but some information has to be reported.

Step 2: Reach the core of the problem

To know about the problem you have to be an excellent listener, a good observer and truly compassionate at heart.

Listen to her without interruption. Do not be in a hurry. Respect her silence. Be attentive also to her body language. Show her nonverbal signs that you are listening like nodding your head.

Ask questions but do not interrogate. Pose questions that are open and allow her to talk. Do not ask questions beginning with "Why".

Allow her to name the feeling underlying her emotions.

Chose your statements wisely. Do not use words to overly dramatize the situation or demean her. Do not label or judge.

Step 3: To know if this has been addressed before and what has been done

When someone discloses violence it has taken her huge courage in doing so. It is quite possible that this is the first time that she wants to talk about it. Women decide to take that path only after they feel they have nothing left to lose and are willing to risk their lives.

It is therefore very important to ensure that the victim has a positive experience when reaching out for help. A poor, slow or inappropriate response may cause a victim to retreat and change their minds about asking for help.

Sometimes abusers apologize to the victims and promise to never use violence again. They begin to hope that violence has ended and that their troubles have passed. They need to be taught to read a man's behaviour and beware. She can trust him but definitely needs to have her alarm on all the time.

Step 4: Educate her

Most of the times women are ignorant. They do not know what exactly can they do about it. Here comes the role of education and awareness. Educate her about the where abouts. Ask her to slowly start building a social support network for herself.

Look for options of housing and work on the finances that will be needed when she will be independent. Encourage her to be independent financially and emotionally. Ask her to look for employment options. By educating her you are in a way preparing her to face her tomorrow in a much stronger way.

Give her information about different national programs, NGOs and institutions that can come to her rescue.

Step 5: Plan of action

Your job does not end by just educating her. Even after giving her all the information she might still not be in a position to make strong decisions mentally. Sit with her and have a plan of action ready when in need. There has to be a stepwise approach to escape. A slow preparation would be a safe rescue. However, she definitely needs to be ready for an emergency escape too.

Discussions on what to do and where to go has to be planned thoroughly well.

A few tips, e.g. for a victim of domestic violence would be:

- All the important documents and keys have to be kept ready in a bag in an easily accesible yet a hidden place.
- She does not need to take all her stuff when leaving. This can be taken later with the help of a police.
- She has to keep her cell phone charged at all times.
- A close neighbour has to be kept in the loop for help in case of an emergency. However, the escape whereabouts need not be disclosed.
- She needs to mentally prepare her kids slowly and wisely.

Step 6: Conclusion of the program

The lady needs to realise that her self respect and safety are of utmost importance. She can bring a change in her life by a thorough plan for doing so.

Structured interactive activities, individual counselling sessions, media (visual or print) therapy, 24-hour helpline and group psychosocial support are a few ways for helping the survivor come out of trauma.

Art therapy has been tried and tested and have shown good results in helping children come out of trauma.

Need of the Hour

There is an urgent need to develop basic minimum standards and procedures for aiding victims of sexual and domestic violence that can be applied in (and are mindful of) varying cultural and social settings. Something which can be truly done and needs a multispeciality involvement is a "One Stop Care", generally located within or connected to a hospital, offers medical and forensic services, psychosocial counseling, legal aid, case management and referrals, and police services on site.

There is also an urgent need to break down the barriers that prevent physicians and other health care providers from providing care to survivors of sexual violence. Some of these barriers include lack of capacity of hospitals/clinics, insufficient resources, cultural barriers, lack of education about the clinical management of rape, confusion and lack of awareness of the 72-hour window for treatment, stigmatization, and laws that require only qualified doctors to provide treatment and documentation that could be provided by properly trained medical personnel.

Safe social spaces can be organized around a physical space such as a community centre or a women's centre where women, adolescent girls and (other) child survivors can go to receive compassionate, caring, appropriate and confidential assistance.

SOURCE REFERENCES AND SUGGESTED READING

1. www.firstaction.eu, Psychosocial support for victims od domestic and gender based violence handbook, First action against violence, cofunded by the rights, equality and citizenship. Programme of the European Union.
2. American Psychiatric Association—Guide to Intimate Partner Violence Among Women, by D Sapkota, published in 2019.
3. https://tpocambodia.org/mental-health-for-survivors-of-gender-based-violence-sexual-assault/

Challenges and Concerns in Young Adult and Adult Survivors of Sexual Assault

Padmaja Samant

Background

There are some societal characteristics, rather shortcomings that we must bear in mind while responding cases of sexual assault/abuse or other forms of violence against women and girls. Gender roles, norms and gender limitations of men and women are well entrenched in the minds of health care providers regardless of their own gender.

The gender roles, norms and gender limitations of men and women are imprinted in the minds and psyche of even the survivors of violence as well as their natal and marital family members.

Gender roles dictate what happens before, during and after assault or abuse to the girls and women at home, in workplaces, in hospitals or clinics in police stations and in the court of law.

So, if we want to change the outcome, we all have to reframe gender-based violence in our own minds.

With this background we shall see some cases that challenge us, frustrate us, weaken our inner voices and blur the logic. Reframing gender will push us and prod us into affirmative advocacy for the survivors.

We should also have a close look at Ministry of Health Guidelines on Response to Sexual Violence to clarify doubts.

Cases

1. A 17-year-old girl was brought by police and her grandfather in advanced pregnancy for obstetric and forensic examination and the needful. The girl was in sound mind, but scared and kept on changing her history. Her parents were not alive and the girl had been brought up by the grandparents. The grandfather was very concerned and protective of the granddaughter and kept saying that an occasional visitor had assaulted her. The girl kept changing her account of the incident. After a lot of counseling, the girl said that after her grandmother's death, the grandfather had been abusing her. When asked why she did not complain earlier, she said that the grandfather had been very kind and affectionate towards the siblings. She felt it was her duty to abide by his wishes. She was also apprehensive about how the extended family would react if she complained against the grandfather. The girl was admitted for social reasons under vigil of a woman police officer. The girl

delivered a live child at term and after sending necessary forensic evidence to the Forensic Science Laboratory (FSL) and the girl and the neonate were sent to a foster home through Child Welfare Committee.

This situation highlights importance of non-judgemental and noncoercive counseling and empathy. The question of autonomy of a minor also arises if she does not consent to examination or reporting to FSL. Generally, the lack of consent is out of fear, ignorance and rarely to protect a love interest. On counseling about short-term and long-term consequences of risky behaviour, the survivors understand and consent to examination.

Importance of teams: The clinician should not need to spend his/her precious time in moving the machinery of police, Child Welfare Committee (CWC) and child protection officers for timely rehabilitation of the survivor and babies born of such assaults. Organisations like Indian Association for Promotion of Adoption and Child Welfare in collaboration with CWC help in rehabilitation of the young people and children in need of shelter.

Differences in wishes of the survivor and her family on whether the child should or should not be given up for adoption is also a matter of concern. Intervention by medical social worker and psychologist is recommended. In this case, paternity testing would give a conclusive verdict; but in case there were no pregnancy, forensic psychologist might be an asset to a multidisciplinary team. The forensic psychologist could help in evaluation and assessment of fabrication and malingering on part of both, the complainant as well as the accused.[1] The challenge is to find such qualified specialists to aid in substantiating the version or statement of the survivor.

2. An adult woman married for about 7 months came with a very unusual complaint. After a few months of marriage and peno-vaginal sexual intercourse her husband started having peno-anal sexual intercourse with her, against her wishes. She stated that after frequent peno-anal sexual intercourse, she started having abdominal pain, constipation and painful defecation. On anal examination by a surgeon anal fissure was diagnosed. The forensic specialist on the team was hesitant to write opinion that the physical complaint and examination findings were attributable to forceful anal penetration. His contention was that abdominal pain and constipation are common complaint and constipation itself can give rise to fissure. He also thought that the offence was hard to prove in the court of law.

In this case, their relation to the compliant and findings to the nature of assault could not be ignored.

We must remember that it is the examining doctor's responsibility to document narration of the survivor/patient of the events in her words as far as possible and to elucidate a plausible explanation for the injuries or findings and their connection to the nature of assault as stated. The courts need a clear opinion of the expert witness (examining physician) to come to a conclusion on the offence.

The words 'alleged history'—though commonplace in medical parlance, also denote deliberate allegation. 'Allegation' and 'Complaint against' evoke different responses from the person taking in the information. 'Stated' or 'Complained' are neutral words and may be used in place of 'Alleged'. An important aspect of writing opinion is being unbiased. So, making possible connection between injuries and the nature of assault as stated only requires logic and experience. Most medical examiners hesitate to write provisional opinion and write 'opinion pending forensic laboratory reports' as they are apprehensive about cross examination. As per the national guidelines on medico-legal care for survivors/victims of sexual violence—'An inference must be drawn in the opinion, correlating the history and clinical findings.'[2]

As per the national guidelines, a registered medical practitioner should be able to examine, document, collect evidence and submit a report to the investigating officer.[2] Hence, it is crucial that all medical graduates are trained in conducting examination, treatment and opinion drafting in cases of sexual assaults of all kinds.

Sexual offences in married couples: There are some socially entrenched notions that make us reluctant to opine on the assault or abuse by a spouse because of a belief that it is the couple's private matter. Marital rape is still not criminalised in India. The exception 2 under Section 375 of Indian Penal Code exempts—forced sexual intercourse by a man with his wife who is over fifteen years of age—from definition of rape. This violates the rights provisions in Article 14 and Article 21 of the Constitution of India. Prof. Sandra Fredman from Oxford University who opined that all levels of the criminal justice system should be provided training to ensure awareness that—**"marriage should not be regarded as extinguishing the legal or sexual autonomy of the wife"**.[3] There could not be a more eloquent feminist critique on this issue.

3. A woman came with a complaint of voyeurism against her own husband. On learning about the wife's premarital affair, the husband ordered her to have sexual intercourse with the ex boyfriend in (husband's) own presence.

   What sort of crime is this? And who should undergo examination? What evidence may be collected and what could be expected in examination findings?

   Since neither force nor resistance may be involved in such a case, injures are unlikely to be found. The physician's job is only to document history and findings and if the woman comes early enough after the sexual Act, necessary swabs may be collected to prove the source of genetic material (semen). Still, the proving of voyeuristic crime of the husband is beyond physical examination of the survivor.

   Nevertheless, opinion cannot be denied.

   Reason for lack of physical and genital findings and possible lack of genetic material should be stated in clear terms. A physician's job is to clarify in the court the possible reasons for presence or absence of injuries and limitations of physical examination in such cases.

   Also a comment on mental state of the survivor by the psychiatrist on the team may clarify her fear, anxiety and helplessness to the court. In this case too, role of forensic psychologist is very crucial in evaluation and assessment of fabrication and malingering on part of both the partners and evaluation of voyeuristic disorder of the accused.

4. An unmarried adult woman came with complaint of sexual assault by a distant relative when she had visited his house for a family function. The survivor was a sexually active person. She had also undergone a medical termination of pregnancy in the past.

   On examination, she had no injuries on private parts and no physical injuries as she was afraid to resist.

   In such a case, it is important to word the opinion giving explanation for lack of injury.

Should one write about the past sexual history? Will it work for or against her? These are the dilemmas in the mind of the physician. In this case, past sexual history could help clarify lack of injuries.

Consensual pre-marital sex by an adult is not a crime. It is prudent to not let moral beliefs come in the way of appropriate documentation.

5. An adult woman with subnormal intelligence was brought by parents with advanced (third trimester) pregnancy (not for assault investigation but for obstetric care). According to the patient the sex was consensual. After delivery the woman and her parents expressed a wish to take the child home.

    Should a police case be done?

    Can the parents of the woman be allowed to take the child home?

    With subnormal intelligence a woman is likely to be chronically sexually abused. Determination of intelligence quotient should be undertaken by the psychologist or psychiatrist on the multidisciplinary team. If unavailable, one can be invited on case to case basis with the help of appropriate authority. In case of women with special needs, special educators and interpreters are also available through the gender resource centre of Mumbai Municipal Corporation.

    Such complex cases are heard by CWC and decisions regarding custody of the newborn and rehabilitation of the survivor are reached. Cases registered with the CWC are also kept under surveillance to prevent child trafficking.

CONCLUSION

Sexual assault and abuse are complex crimes where interagency cooperation is crucial. Administrative support goes a long way in achieving speedy rehabilitation.

Achieving understanding of gender dimensions of crimes, empathy and educating oneself on testifying in the court are important for each health care provider to do justice to his/her job.

It is recommended that all postgraduate trainees in gynaecology and obstetrics as well as paediatrics should familiarise themselves with the procedure of examination and documentation of sexual assault.

Manual for Medical Examination of Sexual Assault by CEHAT is a recommended reading and a ready-reckoner especially while doing age determination, dating injuries. The national guidelines should be read by all trainees to familiarise themselves with interagency cooperation and interface.

REFERENCES

1. https://www.thechicagoschool.edu/insight/psychology/forensic-psychology-sexual-assault/
2. https://main.mohfw.gov.in/reports/guidelines-and-protocols-medico-legal-care-survivors-victims-sexual-violence.
3. Justice Verma Committee Report Summary | RSIndiawww.prsindia.org › report-summaries › justice-verma-committee.

Helplines for Survivors

Reena J Wani, Arvind B Mulay

Background

Domestic and sexual violence has been described as the hidden pandemic within the COVID pandemic, but it is only the tip of the iceberg due to low reporting. Rape is the fourth most common crime against women in India. The government also classifies consensual sex committed on the false promise of marriage as rape. The willingness to report rapes have increased in recent years, after several incidents received widespread media attention and triggered local and nationwide public protests. This led the government to reform its penal code for crimes of rape and sexual assault. All these aspects have been discussed in the earlier sections of this book.

Our Experience

Maharashtra being one of the states with most number of reported sexual assaults against women, perhaps due to increased awareness and work done by NGOs. Mumbai, a bustling metro city and commercial hub, reported the second highest number of crime against women.

In our institute Cooper Hospital, Mumbai, over the period of two years the reported number of sexual assault cases against women were 359 and 265 in 2019 and 2020. The awareness about reporting to hospital or police is increasing day by day due to media and helplines from various NGO and police. The slight decline in numbers in 2020 was probably due to issues of access during lockdown. The efforts are to provide "one stop" crisis centers wherever possible.

KEM Hospital in Mumbai has a 24-hour helpline number for women in distress, both domestic and sexual violence.

We present here some of the available contact numbers, excerpts from KAVACH booklet.

Helplines for Women in Distress

All India	
Central Social Welfare Board—Police Helpline	1091/1291/011-23317004
Shakti Shalini—Women Shelter	011-24373736/7
Saarthak	011-26853846/26524061

Jagori	011-26692700
Joint Women's Programme	011-24619821
Sakshi—Violence Intervention Center	0124-2562336
Saheli	011-24616485
Nirmal Niketan	011-27859158
Nari Raksha Samiti	011-23973949
Rahi	011-26238466/26224042/26227647
Marg	011-26497483/6925
Pratidhi	011-22527259
CATS	1099
CEHAT Emergency number, Mumbai	9029073154
SNEHA, Mumbai One Stop Center at KEM	2224100599
SNEHA Dharavi Helpline, Mumbai	9833052684
SGPRC, Mumbai	9167535765

Women Helpline NGO

All India	
Women Helpline (All India)	1091
National Commission for Women (NCW)	011-26942369, 26944754
Andhra Pradesh	
National Commission for Women	011-13237166
Women Protection Cell	040-23320539
Women Police Station	040-27853508
AP Women's Network	040-27014394
Hyderabad Women Police Station	040-27852400/4852
Bihar	
Women Helpline Centre	18003456247/0612-2320047/2214318
Women Commission	0612-2507800
Bangalore	
Women's Police Helpline, Bangalore (Vanitha Sahayavani)	080-22943225
Bangalore Traffic Police	080-22868444/22868550
Chandigarh	
Women Police Exchange	0172-2741900
Women Helpline	0172-2741900, 1091
Samvad	0172-2546389
Chennai/Tamil Nadu	
Women Helpline	1091

Delhi	
Delhi Commission for Women (DCW)	011-23378044/23378317/23370597
Women Protection Cell	011-24673366/4156/7699
Central Social Welfare Board	1091/1291 (011) 23317004
Outer Delhi Helpline	011-27034873, 27034874
Women in Distress	1091
Police Control Room	100
Child Helpline	1098
Anti Stalking/Obscene Calls	1096
Child, Student and Senior Citizen	1291
DCP, SN Mosobi, North East Special Unit	9818099070
IGP, Robin Hibu, Nodal Officer for Northeasterners	(Whatsapp no)-9810083486
Gujarat	
Women Helpline	1091
Ahmedabad Women's Action Group	079-27470036
Self Employed Women's Association	079-25506477/25506444
The Abhyam Women Helpline	181
Haryana	
Women and Child Helpline	0124-2335100
Haryana Women Commission	0172-2584039, 0172-2583639
Helpline for Women in Distress	9911599100
Himachal Pradesh	
Women's Commission	981606642, 09418636326 09816882491, 9418384215
Karnataka	
Women Police Helpline	0821-2418400
Mysore Women Police Station	0821-2418110/2418410
Women Helpline Number	080-22942149, 1091
Women Commission	080-22100435/22862368, 080-2216485
Kerala	
Women Police Helpline (Trivandrum)	9995399953
State Vanitha Cell	0471-2338100
Women's Cell, Kollam	0474-2742376
Women's Cell, Kochi	0484-2396730
Women Helpline	1091
Kerala Women's Commission	0471-2322590, 2320509, 2337589, 2339878, 2339882

Kolkata	
Women Helpline	1091
Madhya Pradesh	
SP Office/We Care For You	0731-2522111
Mahila Thana	0731-2434999
Pardeshipura	0731-2435999
Sanyogitaganj	0731-2523999
Pandrinath	0731-2342999
Mari Mata (Banganga)	0731-2423999
Juni Indore	0731-2362999
MIG	0731-2570111
Mallharganj	0731-2454201
Women Commission	0755-2661813, 2661802, 2661806
Maharashtra	
Majlis	022-26661252/26662394
Women Right Initiative	022-43411603/43411604
Human Rights Law Network	022-23439754/23436692
Mumbai Police Women Helpline	022-22633333, 22620111
Maharashtra Women Helpline	022-26111103, 1298, 103
Stree Aadhar Kendra	022-24394104/24394103
Mumbai	
Railway Police	9833331111
Mumbai Police Helpline	100, 103
Navi Mumbai Police Station	022-27580255
Pune	
Women Helpline	1091
Punjab	
Women Helpline	9781101091
Women Commission	0172-2712607
Samvad	0172-2546389, 2700109, 276000114
Rajasthan	
Women Helpline	0141-2744000
Nirbhaya Sambhali Helpline	1800-1200-020
Women Police Station, Jodhpur	0291-2012112
Women Commission	0141-2779001-4

Tamil Nadu

Women Commission	044-28551155
Snehdi	044-2446293
The Banyan	044-26530504/26530105
Women Helpline	044-28592750
Women Police Station, Adayar	044-24415732, 044-23452586
Women Police Station, Guindy	044-24700011

Tripura

Commission for Women	0381-2323355, 2322912

Uttar Pradesh

Sahyog NGO	0522-2341319, 2310747
Vanangana	05198-236985
Aali	0522-2782066/60
Women Commission	0522-2306403, 18001805220

West Bengal

Women Commission	91-33-23595609, 91-33-23210154, 91-33-2217 4019/2244 8092
Swayam	033-24863367/3368/3357
Women Helpline Number	033-23595609, 23210154

Goa

Women Helpline	1091, 0832-2421208
Women Commission	0832-2421080

Assam

Women Helpline	181, 9345215029, 0361-2521242
Women Commission	0361-2227888, 2220150, 0361-2220013

Arunachal Pradesh

Women Commission	0360-2214567

Chhattisgarh

Women Commission (Gaytri Bhawan, 13 Jalvihar Colony, Raipur)	0771-2429977, 4013189 18002334299, 0771-4241400

Women Helpline NGO

All India	
All India Women Conference	011-23389680/1165
SNEHA	9833052684/9167535765
Jagori	011-26692700
Saarthak	011-26853846/26524061

Nari Raksha Samiti	011-23973949
Lawyers Collective Womens Rights (Domestic Voilence Cases)	011-24373993/2923
Pratidhi (Legal help)	011-22527259
Sewa	011-25841369/079-25506444
Snehalaya	0241-2778353
NEN (North East Network)	9435017824
Azad Foundation	011-40601878
CREA	011-24378701
CSR (Centre for Social Research)	011-26125583
Vimochana	080-25492781
Swaniti	9821959901
Makam	020-25880786
Janodaya	080-23557777
Aasra	022-27546669
Swayam	033-24863367
Bharatiya Grameen Mahila Sangh	011-46643333
Sayfty	9335037018
Care India	0120-4048250
Swayam	9830772814
Tara Women Centre	080-25251929
Nava Karnataka Mahila Rakshana Vedike	9490135167
Abhayashrama	080-22220834
Vimochana	080-25492781
Samaja Seva Samithi	080-26600022
Vanitha Sahayavani	080-22943225
Shakti Shalini	011-24373736/7
Girls Count	9654445452
Educate Girls	9999372857
Mamta	7774906147
UNICEF	9314039428
Aridhima Medical Education and Research Society	7726020908
Praveen Lata Sansthan	0141-2630526/9828096801/9828455268
UNFPA	9828455268
Plan India	9460209399
SRKPS	9414080218
Pravah Jaipur Initiative	9610009333/8302485842
Save the Children	9828064168

Bharti Foundation	9910604383
Vaagdhara	9414102643
Antakshari Foundation	9413340966
SSSPR	9828163831
PCCRCS	9887068869
Gayatri Seva Sansthan	9983327304
Ashra Vikas Sansthan	9828242855
Shrushti Seva Sansthan	8890272733
Aravali	9414193151
Urmul Sansthan	9414137093
FXB Suraksha India	8860221098
ARIHR	9460387130
IPE Global	9560992047
CRY	9899110837
AAA	9414022032
Amied Alwar	9413304746
Cuts CHD, Chittorgarh	9829143632
Prayas, Chittorgarh	9414110328
Navachar, Chittorgarh	9413315713
CHEER, Jaipur	9983469760
Prayatan	9414028004
Cecoedecon	7389927099
Bodh Shiksha Samiti	9829018460
UN Women	9582803939
Tabaar	8426041518
Vikalp	9414146408
IDS	9829067476
CFAR	8003590301
SNVS, Bharatpur	7976175664
Unnayan Samiti	9530153078
IIFL	9029358815
Impact	9982001816
Jeevan Ashram	9251638751
Umang	9928387735
CDAR	9414059848
Digantar	9414074231
Foster Care Society	9414029147
Freedom Fund	9414066564

Pratham	9351414259
RIHR	9460387130
CCP	9414843654
Independent Thought	9971884900
World Vision India	9907033245
SARATHI Trust	9694426078
WASCO	02969-233150
Manjari Sansthan	9829096288
Population Foundation of India	9928566576
Muskan	9001390064
Jatan Sanathan	9166633337/9950817188
Astha Sansthan	0294-2451348

 Kindly scan the QR code or visit link for Helplines available for women in distress in Maharashtra **http://standupagainstviolence.org/en_US/maharashtra/#mumbai**

CONCLUSION

With the changing times women should not be afraid of contacting NGOs, police or authorities for the help against harassment, domestic or sexual assault. As we all know suffering torture is also labelled as a kind of cowardice, but women may not know where to go, hence do not speak up.

This compilation is an attempt to prepare a list which can help women to speak up against assaults and make our country truly independent.

Acknowledgements

The KAVACH Booklet with details of Laws, phone apps and helplines was prepared with inputs of Sun Senora Team guided by their GM Dr Rashmi Parekh, and has been circulated at various public forums and workshops.

This was released in 2020 by FOGSI President Dr Alpesh Gandhi and Team.

The full version is available on website www.fogsi.org

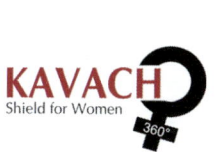

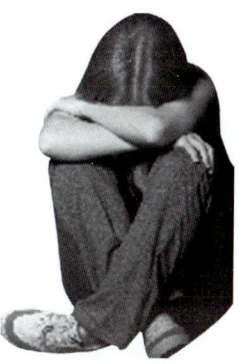

Medico-legal Examination Report of Sexual Violence

1. Name of the Hospital .... OPD No. .... Inpatient No ....
2. Name .... D/o or S/o (where known).......................................
3. Address...
4. Age (as reported) .... Date of Birth (if known)..............................
5. Sex (M/F/Others) ....
6. Date and Time of arrival in the hospital ....
7. Date and Time of commencement of examination...
8. Brought by... (Name & signatures)
9. MLC No. ....Police Station...................................
10. Whether conscious, oriented in time and place and person..............................
11. Any physical/intellectual/psychosocial disability ....

(Interpreters or special educators will be needed where the survivor has special needs such as hearing/speech disability, language barriers, intellectual or psychosocial disability.)

12. Informed Consent/refusal

I...D/o or S/o...
hereby give my consent for:

a) medical examination for treatment   Yes ☐   No ☐
b) this medico-legal examination   Yes ☐   No ☐
c) sample collection for clinical & forensic examination   Yes ☐   No ☐

I also understand that as per law the hospital is required to inform police and this has been explained to me.

I want the information to be revealed to the police   Yes ☐   No ☐

I have understood the purpose and the procedure of the examination including the risk and benefit, explained to me by the examining doctor. My right to refuse the examination at any stage and the consequence of such refusal, including that my medical treatment will not be affected by my refusal, has also been explained and may be recorded. Contents of the above have been explained to me in .... language with the help of a special educator/interpreter/support person (circle as appropriate) ....

If special educator/interpreter/support person has helped, then his/her name and signature...............

Name & signature of survivor or parent/guardian/person in whom the child reposes trust in case of child (<12 years)

....

....

....

With date, time & place
Name & signature/thumb impression of Witness

....

....

....

With date, time & place

13. Marks of identification (any scar/mole)

(1) ....

(2) ....

Left Thumb impression

14. Relevant medical/surgical history

Onset of menarche (in case of girls)   Yes/No   Age of onset..............................

Menstrual history — cycle length and duration .... last menstrual period.............

Menstruation at the time of incident — Yes/No, Menstruation at the time of examination —Yes/ No

Was the survivor pregnant at time of incident — Yes/No, if yes duration of pregnancy ....
weeks

Contraception use: Yes/No....... if yes —method used: ....

Vaccination status— tetanus (vaccinated/not vaccinated), hepatitis B (vaccinated/not vaccinated)

15 A.History of sexual violence

(I) Date of incident/s being reported	(ii) Time of incident/s	(iii) Location/s

(iv)Estimated duration : 1–7 days…….. 1 week to 2 months…………………………………
2–6 months…………….. >6 months……………………………………………………………………………….
Episode: One…………. Multiple …….…..…Chronic (>6 months) ……..Unknown……….

(v) Number of assailant(s) and
      name/s…………………….....………………………...…………………………………………
(vi) Sex of assailant(s)…………………….....……………………Approx. Age of assailant(s)
……………………........ If known to the survivor—relationship with the
survivor…..…………………………………………………………………………………..……….

(vii) Description of incident in the words of the narrator:
Narrator of the incident: survivor/informant (specify name and relation to survivor)
………………

If this space is insufficient use extra page

15 B. Type of physical violence used if any (describe)

Hit with (hand, fist, blunt object, sharp object)	Burned with
Biting	Kicking
Pinching	Pulling Hair
Violent shaking	Banging head
	Dragging
Any other:	

15 C.

i.   Emotional abuse or violence if any (insulting, cursing, belittling, terrorizing).........
....

ii. Use of restraints if any ....

iii. Used or threatened the use of weapon(s) or objects if any..............................
....

iv. Verbal threats (for example, threats of killing or hurting survivor or any other person in whom the survivor is interested; use of photographs for blackmailing, etc.) if any:
....

v.   Luring (sweets, chocolates, money, job) if any: ....

vi. Any other:..

15 D.

i.   Any history of drug/alcohol intoxication:

ii. Whether sleeping or unconscious at the time of the incident: ....

15 E. If survivor has left any marks of injury on assailant/s, enter details: ....

15 F. Details regarding sexual violence

Was penetration by penis, fingers or object or other body parts (Write Y=Yes, N=No, DNK=Do not know)?**Mention and describe body part/s and/or object/s used for penetration.**

	Penetration			Emission of semen		
Orifice of victim	By penis	By body part of self or assailant or third party (finger, tongue or any other)	By object	Yes	No	Do not know
Genitalia (vagina and/or urethra)						
Anus						
Mouth						

Oral sex performed by assailant on survivor	Y	N	DNK
Forced masturbation of self by survivor	Y	N	DNK
Masturbation of assailant by survivor, forced manipulation of genitals of assailant by survivor	Y	N	DNK
Exhibitionism (perpetrator displaying genitals)	Y	N	DNK
Did ejaculation occur outside body orifice (vagina/anus/mouth/urethra)?	Y	N	DNK

If yes, describe where on the body			
Kissing, licking or sucking any part of survivor's body	Y	N	If yes, describe
Touching/fondling	Y	N	If yes, describe
Condom used*	Y	N	DNK
If yes status of condom	Y	N	DNK
Lubricant used*	Y	N	DNK
If yes, describe kind of lubricant used			
If object used, describe object:			
Any other forms of sexual violence			

* Explain what condom and lubricant is to the survivor

Post incident has the survivor	Yes/No/Do not know	Remarks
Changed clothes Changed undergarments Cleaned/washed clothes Cleaned/washed undergarments Bathed Douched Passed urine Passed stools Rinsing of mouth/brushing/vomiting (circle any or all as appropriate)		

Time since incident.. H/o vaginal/anal/oral bleeding/discharge prior to the incident of sexual violence...................

History of vaginal/anal/oral bleeding/discharge since the incident of sexual violence.......

History of painful urination/ painful defecation/ fissures/ abdominal pain/pain in genitals or any other part since the incident of sexual violence

16. General physical examination
i.   Is this the first examination..
ii. Pulse....................................... BP..
iii. Temp...Resp. rate......................................
iv. Pupils ....
v.   Any observation in terms of general physical wellbeing of the survivor....................

17. Examination for injuries on the body if any

The pattern of injuries sustained during an incident of sexual violence may show considerable variation. This may range from complete absence of injuries (more frequently) to grievous injuries (very rare).

(Look for bruises, physical torture injuries, nail abrasions, teeth bite marks, cuts, lacerations, fracture, tenderness, any other injury, boils, lesions, discharge specially on the scalp, face, neck, shoulders, breast, wrists, forearms, medial aspect of upper arms, thighs and buttocks) Note the injury type, site, size, shape, colour, swelling signs of healing (simple/grievous, dimensions.)

Scalp examination for areas of tenderness (if hair pulled out/ dragged by hair)	
Facial bone injury: Orbital blackening, tenderness	
Petechial haemorrage in eyes and other places	
Lips and buccal mucosa / gums	
Behind the ears	
Eardrum	
Neck, shoulders and breast	
Upper limb	
Inner aspect of upper arms	
Inner aspect of thighs	
Lower limb, buttocks	
Other, please specify	

Right   Left

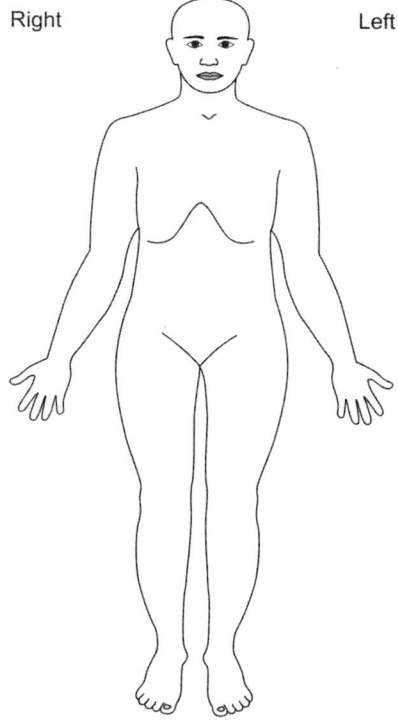

Figure A1

Right   Left

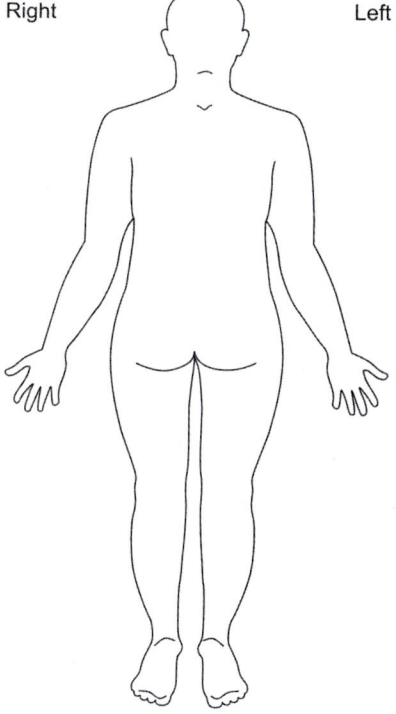

Figure A2

18. Local examination of genital parts/other orifices*

A. External genitalia: Record findings and state NA where not applicable.

Body parts to be examined	Findings	
Urethral meatus & vestibule		
Labia majora		
Labia minora		
Fourchette & introitus		
Hymen perineum		
External urethral meatus		
Penis		
Scrotum		
Testes		
Clitoropenis		
Labioscrotum		
Any other		

* Per vaginum /per speculum examination should not be done unless required for detection of injuries or for medical treatment.

P/S findings if performed ....
P/V findings if performed ....
Record reasons if P/V of P/S examination performed ....

C. Anus and rectum (encircle the relevant)
Bleeding/ tear/ discharge/ oedema/ tenderness

D. Oral cavity (encircle the relevant)
Bleeding/ discharge/ tear/oedema/ tenderness

19. Systemic examination

Central nervous System: ....
Cardiovascular system: ....
Respiratory system: ....
Chest: ....
Abdomen: ....

Right   Left

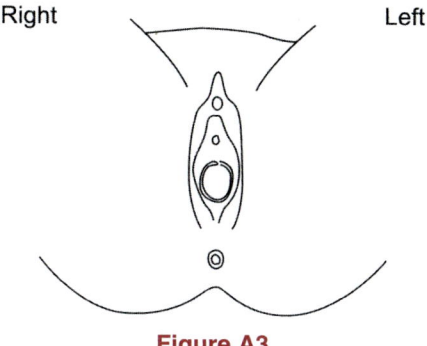

Figure A3

Right   Left

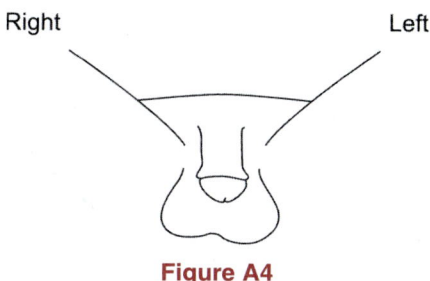

Figure A4

Right   Left

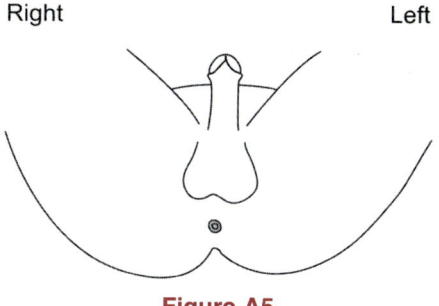

Figure A5

20. Sample collection/investigations for hospital laboratory/clinical laboratory

1) Blood for HIV, VDRL, HbsAg
2) Urine test for pregnancy
3) Ultrasound for pregnancy/internal injury
4) X-ray for Injury

21. Samples Collection for Central/ State Forensic Science Laboratory

1) Debris collection paper
2) Clothing evidence where available (to be packed in separate paper bags after air drying)

List and details of clothing worn by the survivor at time of incident of sexual violence

3) Body evidence samples as appropriate (duly labeled and packed separately)

	Collected/ not collected	Reason for not collecting
Swabs from stains on the body (blood, semen, foreign material, others)		
Scalp hair (10–15 strands)		
Head hair combing		
Nail scrapings (both hands separately)		
Nail clippings (both hands separately)		
Oral swab		
Blood for grouping, testing drug/alcohol intoxication (plain vial)		
Blood for alcohol levels (sodium fluoride vial)		
Blood for DNA analysis (EDTA vial)		
Urine (drug testing)		
Any other (tampon/sanitary napkin/condom/object)		

4) **Genital and anal evidence** (each sample to be packed, sealed, and labeled separately—to be placed in a bag)

* Swab sticks for collecting samples should be moistened with distilled water provided.

	Collected/ not collected	Reason for not collecting
Matted pubic hair		
Pubic hair combing (mention if shaved)		
Cutting of pubic hair (mention if shaved)		
Two vulval swabs (for semen examination and DNA testing)		
Two vaginal swabs (for semen examination and DNA testing)		
Two anal swabs (for semen examination and DNA testing)		
Vaginal smear (air-dried) for semen examination		
Vaginal washing		
Urethral swab		
Swab from glans of penis/clitoropenis		

*Samples to be preserved as directed till handed over to police along with duly attested sample seal.

22. Provisional medical opinion

I have examined (name of survivor)..............M/F/Other.................aged.............................
reporting_ (type of sexual violence and circumstances)..................., XYZ days/hours after the incident, after having (bathed/douched, etc.)..................... My findings are as follows:

• Samples collected (for FSL), awaiting reports
• Samples collected (for hospital laboratory)
• Clinical findings
• Additional observations (if any)

23. Treatment prescribed

Treatment	Yes	No	Type and comments
STI prevention treatment			
Emergency contraception			
Wound treatment			
Tetanus prophylaxis			
Hepatitis B vaccination			
Post-exposure prophylaxis for HIV			
Counselling			
Other			

24. Date and time of completion of examination ....

This report contains .... number of sheets and .... number of envelopes.

Signature of Examining Doctor

Name of Examining Doctor

Place: Seal

25. Final opinion (after receiving laboratory reports)

Findings in support of the above opinion, taking into account the history, clinical examination findings and laboratory reports of .... bearing identification marks described above, ... hours/days after the incident of sexual violence, I am of the opinion that:

Signature of Examining Doctor

Name of Examining Doctor

Place: Seal

COPY OF THE ENTIRE MEDICAL REPORT MUST BE GIVEN TO THE SURVIVOR/ VICTIM FREE OF COST IMMEDIATELY

Glossary of Terms

BPR & D	Bureau of Police Development and Research
CBT	Cognitive Behavioural Therapy
CEDAW	Committee on Elimination of Discrimination Against Women
CEHAT	Centre for Enquiry into Health and Allied Themes
CLA	The Criminal Law (Amendment) Act (Nirbhaya Act)
CMO	Chief Medical Officer
CRC	Convention of the Rights of the Child
CRPD	Convention on the Rights of Persons with Disabilities
CSA	Child Sex Abuse
DAR	District Armed Reserve
DC	District Commissioner
DEVAM	United Nations Declaration on the Elimination of Violence Against Women
DLSA	District Legal Service Authority
DPO	District Programme Officer
DSP	Deputy Superintendent of Police
DVA	Domestic Violence Act
DWDA	District Women's Development Agency
ECP	Emergency Contraception
EMDR	Eye Movement Desensitization and Reprocessing
FIR	First Information Report
FSL	Forensic Science Laboratory
GBV	Gender-Based Violence
HCP	Health Care Provider
ICC	Internal Complaints Committee
ICESCR	International Covenant on Economic, Social and Cultural Rights
IMF	International Monetary Fund
IO	Investigating Officer
IPC	Indian Penal Code
LCC	Local Complaints Committee
LGBT	Lesbian, Gay, Bisexual and Transgender
LNG	Levonorgestrel

MCGM	Municipal Corporation of Greater Mumbai
MoHFW	Ministry of Health and Family Welfare, Union of India
MTP	Medical Termination of Pregnancy
NCPCR	National Commission for Protection of Child Rights
NCW	National Commission for Women
NFHS	National Family Health Survey
NGO	Non-Governmental Organizations
OSC	One Stop Centre
PDS	Public Distribution System
PEP	Post-Exposure Prophylaxis
PFO	Police Facilitation Officer
PG	Postgraduate
PHC	Primary Health Centre
PIL	Public Interest Litigation
PO	Protection Officer
POCSO	The Protection of Children from Sexual Offences
PPR	Police per lakh Population Ratio
PTSD	Post-Traumatic Stress Disorder
PWDVA	Protection of Women Against Domestic Violence Act
RMP	Registered Medical Practitioner
RTS	Rape Trauma Syndrome
SAFE Kit	Sexual Assault Forensic Evidence collection Kit
SLSA	State Legal Service Authority
SNEHA	Society for Nutrition, Education & Health Action
SP	Suprintendent of Police
TOP	Termination of Pregnancy
UNFPA	United Nations Population Fund
UNICEF	United Nations Children's Fund
VAW	Violence Against Women
WDP	Women's Development Project
WHO	World Health Organization

Index